1993

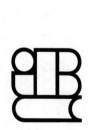

GOVERNING COMMUNITY HOSPITALS

JOHN P. McCOMB, JR.

GOVERNING COMMUNITY HOSPITALS

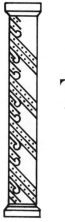

A Primer for Trustees and Health Care Executives

Jossey-Bass Publishers · San Francisco

For sales outside the United States contact Maxwell Macmillan International Publishing Group, 866 Third Avenue, New York, New York 10022

Manufactured in the United States of America

The paper used in this book is acid-free and meets the State of California requirements for recycled paper (50 percent recycled waste, including 10 percent postconsumer waste), which are the strictest guidelines for recycled paper currently in use in the United States.

Library of Congress Cataloging-in-Publication Data

McComb, John P., date.
    Governing community hospitals : a primer for trustees and health care executives / John P. McComb, Jr.—1st ed.
       p.   cm.—(Jossey-Bass health series)
    Includes bibliographical references and index.
    ISBN 1-55542-440-6
    1. Hospitals—Administration. 2. Hospitals—Trustees.   I. Title.
II. Series.
    [DNLM: 1. Governing Board. 2. Hospitals, Community—organization & administration—United States.   WX 150 M479g]
RA971.M42   1992
362.1'1'068—dc20
DNLM/DLC
for Library of Congress   92-2939
                                       CIP

The epigraph at the beginning of the book is from an address given by Rosemary A. Stevens at the American Hospital Association Annual Meeting in July 1990. It is reprinted with her permission.

FIRST EDITION
HB Printing   10 9 8 7 6 5 4 3 2 1   *Code 9241*

The Jossey-Bass Health Series

To my wife, Nan,
for her years of unfailing love,
humor, and support

Contents

Preface

Health care is, and probably will continue to be, the number one domestic policy issue in this country. Involved are conflicting concerns for human health and longevity versus increasing costs and tax liability.

When Medicare was adopted a generation ago, Americans believed that if the federal government paid for something, it was free. But twenty-five years of painfully escalating health care costs have convinced us that there is no free lunch. More than thirty million Americans have been excluded from the system because of their inability to pay. We must find a way to include these people in the system and make it affordable for those who are already covered. Many problems must be solved to sufficiently reduce costs so that we can achieve these goals.

If hospital governing boards have the ultimate legal and moral responsibility for everything that goes on in their institutions, do they have a role in the solution of these problems? This question cannot really be answered until we have a better view of the role and function of these boards at the institutional level. This book should provide such a view.

Hospital trustees have traditionally been educated through the time-consuming and inexact process of on-the-job training. This consists of attending board and committee meetings, listening to presentations by management and by other board members, and gradually assimilating enough information about the hospital to be able to make informed judgments on matters presented to the board for its consideration. This process worked reasonably well when the environment was less complicated, change took place at a slower pace, and public expectations of trustee accountability were less pressing. But many hospitals have begun to limit the length of board tenures to a fixed number of terms. This limited tenure and the slow pace of on-the-job training have lessened the length of useful service of board members at such institutions. A more expeditious and precise system obviously should be developed. Failing that, the present system can be accelerated by taking advantage of educational programs offered by the American Hospital Association (AHA), various state hospital associations, and organizations such as the Estes Park Institute, Volunteer Trustees of Not-for-Profit Hospitals, Charles Ewell's Governance 100, and John Horty's National Conference of Community Hospitals.

Audience

Governing Community Hospitals was written primarily to enable hospitals to establish formal instructional programs for their trustees, to bring new board members quickly up to speed, and to ensure that all board members, new and old, have available to them the knowledge they need to be able to fulfill their responsibilities.

In addition to being a resource for hospital trustees, this book should prove useful in an academic setting by providing a survey course for newcomers to the study of health care. In the spring of 1990, with Samuel A. Friede, a vice president of Shadyside Hospital and Fellow of the American College of Healthcare Executives, I taught a course on hospital governance on an experimental basis in the Graduate School of Public Health at the University of Pittsburgh. A draft of *Governing Community Hospitals* was used as the course syllabus and proved to be a useful guide for classroom instruction. The course has since been added to the school's regular curriculum.

Administrators and managers, including CEOs and CFOs, making a change from the investor-owned to the nonprofit field will find the book useful in helping them to acclimate to the new corporate setting. Their counterparts already in the nonprofit field will find material that has not previously been available to them in one place with respect to nonprofit board responsibilities and potential liability. Students of health care, public health, and health care administration should find the text helpful.

This book should also be useful for managers making the transition from employment in another business field to hospital employment and for corporate employee benefit managers and members of their support staffs who are responsible for corporate decisions affecting the purchase of employee health care. Physicians practicing in the hospital environment or having medical staff or hospital administrative responsibilities need to be familiar with the organizational and operational aspects of community hospitals that the book covers.

Overview of the Contents

Chapter One discusses the present crisis in health care and various plans for its resolution. The plans discussed represent a cross section of reform proposals that have received national attention.

Chapter Two reviews the historical development of the hospital as an institution and the responsibility eventually imposed on trustees for the quality of patient care. The unique organizational structure of the modern hospital is discussed in comparison with that of other organizations.

Chapter Three describes the role of the board and its chair and the distinctions between governance and management. It develops the concept that the board serves as proxy for the community in governing the hospital.

Voluntarism and the nature of the nonprofit corporation are the subject of Chapter Four, which also discusses some recent criticisms of the nonprofit corporation as a vehicle for hospital operation.

Chapter Five is devoted to the recruitment and retention of the chief executive officer and includes suggestions on how to conduct an executive search and evaluate a chief executive officer's performance.

Chapter Six explains how the board works through its committees and how the board periodically evaluates its own performance. A step-by-step self-evaluation process is recommended.

A discussion of objective standards for trustee performance and of various legal, statutory, and regulatory limitations on board discretion is contained in Chapter Seven. This chapter includes a very brief introduction to the antitrust laws.

Chapter Eight concerns trustee responsibility for planning and marketing. It examines the merits and hazards of advertising campaigns in support of the marketing function.

Chapter Nine details trustee accountability for corporate assets. It includes a discussion of hospital accounting and the various third-party reimbursement systems presently in use.

The board's concerns for quality and the question of how the board relates to the organized medical staff are discussed in Chapter Ten, which also includes material on staff organization and credentialing.

Chapter Eleven describes the process of restructuring and its problems, including its potential for adversely affecting public perceptions of community hospitals.

Chapter Twelve covers multihospital systems, alliances, HMOs, PPOs, and other managed care systems. HMOs and PPOs are suggested as the preferred entities for health care delivery in the future.

Finally, Chapter Thirteen contains the author's conclusions and suggestions to trustees for resolving the health care crisis, which include institution-specific strategic planning.

Acknowledgments

In the preparation of this book, Susan Beneman of the Hospital Trustee Association of Pennsylvania has been an invaluable friend and supporter. In addition to providing helpful critical comments, she passed on an early draft to James Redman of Heidrick and Struggles, the executive recruiting firm. He sent me a lengthy letter setting forth a number of very helpful suggestions, which I adopted. Both of these individuals have been helpful throughout.

A draft of the text was submitted to several consultants in the governance field. Sandra Gill of Physician Management Resources and Winifred Hageman of The Umbdenstock-Hageman Partnership responded with detailed critical comments, while Barry Bader of Bader & Associates and James Orlikoff of Orlikoff & Associates were more general in their responses but nonetheless very helpful.

Beaufort Longest, director of the Health Policy Institute at the University of Pittsburgh's Graduate School of Public Health, has also been very helpful.

Buchanan Ingersoll, my law firm, has been very supportive. Virginia A. DeMarco, a trial lawyer, took editorial charge of the project. Daniel Amidon, Vivian Frye, Patricia J. Marley, and Stanley Milavec, all of whom practice in the health care field, reviewed the substance of the book and suggested revisions. Patricia was particularly helpful in this regard. My secretary, Leslie Wright, assisted by Sheryl Gluz and Mickie Fiorillo, has prepared the text and, with Virginia, has coordinated the combined efforts of the firm.

Hope Hudson, a law student at the University of Pittsburgh, working with Virginia, organized the Notes at the end of the book. Thomas E. Boyle, cochairman of the health law section at Buchanan Ingersoll, provided encouragement and support.

The book has been very strongly influenced by my experience as a trustee of Shadyside Hospital in Pittsburgh over a period of thirty-four years. At Shadyside, I have had the invaluable assistance of Mark Scott, treasurer and chief financial officer, who prepared the Pillhaven financial statements in Chapter Nine. Mark also reviewed and edited Chapter Nine. I incorporated a number of changes in the text suggested by Samuel Friede in connection with our teaching collaboration at the University of Pittsburgh. Wendy Lomicka, director of Hospital Relations and Communications, has given me suggestions about book design. The cheerful assistance of Margaret Codispoti and Melinda Fetkovich in the hospital's James Frazer Hillman Health Sciences Library and of Edward Ehrhardt, Jr., director of Corporate Risk Management and senior hospital counsel, are greatly appreciated. Although I have received help from these and many other people, I wish to acknowledge that the responsibility for any errors is mine.

The publisher submitted a draft of the book to Dean C. Coddington, one of the authors of *The Crisis in Health Care: Costs, Choices, and Strategies,* cited in the text. His searching review resulted in many revisions to the book as finally written.

Englewood, Florida   John P. McComb, Jr.
February 1992

The Author

John P. McComb, Jr., (1922–1992) was of counsel to the Pittsburgh law firm of Buchanan Ingersoll and was formerly chairman of its health care law section. He received his B.A. degree (1944) from Princeton University cum laude and, following service in the Marine Corps, received his LL.B. degree (1948), subsequently changed to J.D. (1969), from Harvard Law School. Mr. McComb practiced law independently and as resident counsel for a local investment firm before joining Moorhead & Knox, a law firm that was later merged into Buchanan Ingersoll.

Mr. McComb's law practice involved representation of several hospitals and many other health care institutions. He served, at various times, as vice president of the board of directors of Pittsburgh's Eye & Ear Hospital and as an incorporator and director of the University Health Center of Pittsburgh. In 1958, he was elected a trustee of Shadyside Hospital, and he acted as chairman of that hospital's board from 1984 to 1987.

Mr. McComb served as a trustee of the Hospital Association of Pennsylvania and as a director of the Hospital Trustee Association of Pennsylvania. He was the Pennsylvania delegate to the American Hospital Association's Congress of Hospital Trustees and taught at the University of Pittsburgh's Graduate School of Public Health, where he was a member of the adjunct faculty. In 1991, Mr. McComb was named by the American Hospital Association's *Trustee* magazine as "the trustee who made a difference" in the American Hospital Association's Region 2 (New York, New Jersey, and Pennsylvania).

IN MEMORIAM

Shortly before this book was to be published, I was deeply saddened to learn of the passing of the author, John P. McComb, Jr. Given all the health problems that he had battled so gallantly over the past five years, it seemed terribly unfair for John not to see his book in final form. I soon realized, however, that the physical form of the book would have been irrelevant to John. The task he had set out to accomplish he had completed and he could move on to his next.

To better understand *Governing Community Hospitals* or any book, knowledge of the author is often helpful. John was a person of many talents and great dignity. For over forty years, he practiced many aspects of law, including health law (before there even was such a specialty) and First Amendment law. As an attorney, John zealously advocated his clients' interests in a manner that was effective yet unoffensive. John was also a devoted father whose face invariably lit up when discussing the accomplishments of his four children. In his later years, John finally had time to travel the globe, and he particularly relished visiting the land of his forebears, Scotland, and countries where he had spent time while in the Marine Corps.

John's essential characteristic, however, was the depth of his compassion for others. Whether he was dealing with a secretary, a senior partner of a major law firm, or a physician, John treated everyone with dignity and respect. The principal manifestation of his compassion was his utter devotion to Shadyside Hospital and the health care field. He learned compassion, I believe, from his parents; his father, John P. McComb, Sr., was the head of Obstetrics and Gynecology at Shadyside Hospital. John's belief in the importance of providing high-quality, affordable, accessible health care to all is reflected by the thousands of hours he contributed to Shadyside Hospital during his thirty-three years on its board of trustees. Despite suffering serious health problems in his later years, John continued regularly to attend meetings of the boards of Shadyside Hospital, the Hospital Association of Pennsylvania, and numerous other health care organizations. His goal through all of this service was to upgrade our health care delivery system, especially through the nation's voluntary community hospitals. John's wish was for this book to be one more tool that could be used by hospital boards and management to improve their part in the provision of high-quality health care.

Therefore, while I am distressed to have lost a valued partner, peerless mentor, and reliable friend, I am encouraged by the hope that John McComb's book, *Governing Community Hospitals,* will play a role in enhancing our country's health care system.

Pittsburgh, Pennsylvania   Thomas E. Boyle
March 1992

GOVERNING COMMUNITY HOSPITALS

The United States has . . . created an amazing system of hospitals in the twentieth century: huge, disorganized, nervous, ebullient, dedicated, wasteful, technically innovative, luxurious, inegalitarian, daring, competitive, pluralistic, self-contained, and conflict ridden. Hospitals are organizational chameleons. They can be viewed as both charities and businesses, saviors and profligates, heroes and villains, technological successes, and social failures. American hospitals are overwhelmingly nonfederal, but they are subject to more detailed national regulation—micromanagement—than any other hospital system in the world. Yet the hospitals express, too, the all-American virtues of voluntarism and community—vague, patriotic, and flexible as these may be in terms of showing what hospitals do. We are living in a jungle of ideas about what kind of an enterprise this system is.

> —*Rosemary A. Stevens,*
> *address at American Hospital*
> *Association Annual Meeting,*
> *July 1990*

CHAPTER 1

The Crisis
and the Challenge

We are examining the responsibilities of hospital trustees at a time of unprecedented crisis in the health care delivery system. Hospitals in the United States have evolved rapidly during the past century. Nothing, however, can compare with what lies ahead, since many believe that the current crisis in health care will result in revolutionary changes in the next few years. This first chapter is devoted to a discussion of the principal factors responsible for the crisis and the likely results of reform. The final chapter will then examine trustee responsibility in view of these developments.

You can hardly pick up a newspaper without reading about the health care system in chaos. Costs are out of line and are increasing. We spend more per capita for health care than any other nation in the world and yet we have shorter life expectancies and higher infant mortality rates than many other industrialized countries.

Joseph Califano tells us that Chrysler has to pay so much for its employees' health care that it is handicapped in trying to sell its cars competitively with foreign manufacturers.

Although Medicare and Medicaid were established in 1965 as part of President Lyndon Johnson's vision of the "Great Society," thirty-seven million Americans have been

1

excluded from this great society because they cannot afford health insurance or cannot afford adequate health insurance.

There is an emerging sentiment in this country for the adoption of a system that will provide health care for all Americans—universal health coverage—as a matter of right. But to implement universal health coverage without taking other steps to reform the existing system would result in further disastrous cost escalation that may imperil our payment mechanisms.

The Challenge of Universal Health Coverage

Universal health coverage is an ideal that is consistent with American goals as old as the Republic. How can life, liberty, and happiness be pursued if one is suffering from untreated trauma or disease? It is a fundamental tenet of this book that universal access to health care is a worthwhile and compelling national goal. As a corollary, it should be the responsibility of all hospital trustees, as long as they are carrying out their responsibility to preserve the assets of their institutions, to work toward facilitating the reforms to the system that are necessary to meet this goal.

To posit the need for reform is to assume that there are flaws in the system that need to be addressed. There are. These flaws are numerous and are often identified with the interests of strongly entrenched partisan groups. What is one person's flaw is another person's virtue. To achieve the goal of universal health coverage, we must slay some formidable dragons or pay an unconscionable price.

As the health care crisis deepens, discussions of health care will be dominated by the issue of reform.[1] Several different reform bills have been introduced in Congress. Some states, such as New York, California, and Oregon, doubt the practicability of reform at the national level and are formulating reform programs for their own residents. The Pepper Commission, the American Hospital Association, the National Leadership Commission on Health Care, the Heritage Foundation, Physicians for a National Health Program, and many other organizations have submitted plans for health care reform. It is important that trustees understand the basic issues these plans deal with and the prospective scenarios for reform they set forth. They must understand how different scenarios will affect their institutions. They must follow these scenarios as they are implemented and, where appropriate, try to influence the decision of Congress or the state legislature as to plan content. Trustees must also be sure that their hospital has in place a developing strategic plan to enable the institution to get the maximum benefit from the plan as it is ultimately adopted.

Discussing the issues that contribute to the health care crisis is difficult. The issues do not change, but their relative importance does in relationship to the solutions proposed. Nonetheless, the next section will touch on the major factors involved in the crisis and, following that, we will discuss the various scenarios that have been proposed to resolve the problems.

What Is Causing the Crisis?

Although economists disagree about the principal causes of the crisis, it seems safe to say that, with the exception of cost shifting, the causes are largely cost related. These causes include the following:

- General price inflation
- Excess hospital capacity—nationally, 35 percent of community hospital beds are empty
- Duplication of competitive hospital services—redundant facilities and geographical overlap of clinical departments in competing hospitals are common
- Discounts and uncompensated care
- Cost shifting
- Declining inpatient utilization
- An aging population
- Medical intervention that is not cost effective
- Unnecessary and inappropriate care

- Increase in acuity of inpatient care
- More sophisticated (and expensive) technologies
- Excessive administrative costs
- Health plan–mandated benefits
- Excessive malpractice insurance premiums and other malpractice costs
- Restrictions on health care plan membership such as "pre-existing conditions"

Health care providers are subject to the general price inflation that affects the rest of the economy. In recent years, inflation in health care has averaged from two to two and a half times general price inflation.

Excess hospital capacity increases hospital costs substantially. Even if excess beds are not staffed, institutional fixed costs remain the same but have a smaller divisor than if those excess beds were utilized. For this reason, greater saving is produced by completely closing an underutilized institution rather than closing the same number of beds in several different institutions that continue in existence with their fixed costs unabated.

Excess hospital capacity has another tendency to increase costs. Studies of small area variations in medical practice have shown that where excess beds are available, doctors will tend to hospitalize patients who might not have been hospitalized otherwise. Unnecessary hospital use increases with the supply of hospital beds.[2]

Duplication of services follows from the fact that hospital locations were originally selected on a helter-skelter basis that had little to do with providing a geographically uniform service to the public. In the old days, a rich benefactor would donate property on which to build a hospital together with funds to build and equip it. No matter that it was only two trolley stops from County General, the old Smith estate would make a fine site for Smith Memorial, as indeed it once did. Now we are paying the price for not having had a rational geographical plan when our hospital system was developed.

As a hypothetical example, County General and Smith

Memorial now serve the same geographical area. They compete for patients in all clinical areas in which they now have underutilized duplicate services. Could these hospitals agree with each other that each would give up certain clinical services in favor of the other, thus reducing costs to the public? No. This would be a clear per se violation of the antitrust laws, as we will learn in Chapter Seven.

Discounts are a way of life with hospitals. With the exception of indemnity accounts and private payers, hospitals are almost never paid their billed charges. Through arrangements with other payers, hospitals allow discounts from their billed charges or allowable costs. The amount the hospital is contractually entitled to receive from some payers may be less than its cost in providing such services. This is nearly always true in Medicaid cases and arguably true in most Medicare cases. The estimated value of uncompensated care provided by hospitals each year to the uninsured exceeds $10 billion or approximately $10 thousand per licensed hospital bed.[3]

Hospitals in the past ten years have experienced a shift in demand from inpatient to outpatient treatment. This shift has resulted from improved technology, pressure from third-party payers, and changes in reimbursement patterns. New facilities have been constructed for outpatient treatment, and these have turned out to be convenient both for patients and physicians. Early construction of these facilities often failed, however, to anticipate the volume of outpatient surgery that would be generated as more and more complicated procedures were done on an outpatient basis. This meant that more patients would utilize the recovery areas and for longer periods than had been anticipated. When the recovery areas were full, outpatient surgery would have to be shut down even though there were operating rooms available. This is now being corrected by remodeling the facilities and is no longer a major deterrent to the development of outpatient surgery. As outpatient treatment has expanded, its costs have escalated more rapidly than costs of inpatient treatment. This may be a result of the increasing acuity of cases treated on an outpatient basis. It may also be another example of cost shifting.

The age of the population of the United States is increasing. Persons between the ages of sixty-five and seventy-four use three times the hospital resources utilized by younger people, and those over seventy-five use five times as much as those under sixty-five.[4]

Inappropriate or unnecessary procedures may be increasing medical costs substantially. Louis Sullivan, secretary of the Department of Health and Human Services, has estimated such procedures may run as high as 25 percent, while others have made even higher estimates.[5] Medicine is still an art as much as a science, but a 25 percent error does seem to be excessive. This figure should be reduced as more of the population is enrolled in managed care programs, with their prehospitalization review and second opinion procedures. Similarly, the work of the Agency for Health Care Policy and Research, established by the 101st Congress to promote research on medical outcomes and to develop guidelines for medical practice, could be helpful in reducing this source of health care cost.

Largely because of the introduction of prospective payment for Medicare patients (diagnosis-related groups, or DRGs) in 1982 and the development of outpatient treatment facilities, the acuity of illness of inpatients has increased substantially in the past ten years. As a result of this increase in acuity, more of a hospital's resources are utilized in patient treatment than would be the case for a patient less profoundly ill. Acutely ill patients require more medications and laboratory tests, more utilization of technicians and equipment, and more nursing care. These all add materially to the cost of patient care.

The postwar era has seen enormous strides in the development of technology to support medical advances. Heart/pump machines facilitate open heart surgery; microscopic surgical devices permit new procedures in neurosurgery. Lasers speed and simplify eye surgery, and the development of techniques such as computerized tomography (CT) and magnetic resonance imaging (MRI) has advanced medical diagnostic capabilities far beyond those possible with the X-ray machine. Competition among hospitals in recent years has produced a strong desire in each competitor to have the equipment that will enable it to compete favorably. The costs are substantial, and new equipment now in development will be even more expensive. The greater number of MRIs available in this country as compared with Canada partly explains why health care in this country is 30 percent more expensive than in Canada.

Another heavy burden on our health care financial system is its administrative costs. The American system of having many third-party payers providing hundreds of different health insurance plans adds enormously to the cost of the system. According to a study published in the May 2, 1991, issue of the *New England Journal of Medicine,* administrative costs of health care delivery in 1987 reached 23.9 percent of health care spending.[6] Worse, this was a 37 percent increase during the four-year period from 1983 to 1987. According to a report in *Health Letter* in 1991, these administrative costs came to $193 billion.[7] The article continues that the Canadian health care delivery system, which has only one third-party payer—the government—has an administrative expense component that was only 11 percent in 1987. Moreover, it points out that this percentage rate had fallen 4 points between 1983 and 1987. If the United States could achieve the same efficiency, Americans could save enough to provide health care at current per capita rates for all of the more than thirty million Americans who did not have health care in 1990.

To achieve the administrative efficiencies of the Canadian system, it would be necessary to have only one source of payment for patient care and to have those payments made to each provider on a lump sum basis. The present system involves at least 1,500 different health insurance programs, each with its own processing apparatus and eligibility requirements. Billing is on the equivalent of a per bandaid or per aspirin basis.

Converting to a single-payer system would involve slaying one of our most formidable dragons—free enterprise, championed by the insurance industry—and replacing it with that often-maligned old ogre, the government. Nonetheless, Ohio, Colorado, Michigan, Vermont, and California are con-

sidering legislation that would introduce a single-payer system bringing all state residents within coverage of the plan.

Another major cost burdening the health care system is
the tort system of compensating persons injured by medical
malpractice. Based on state law, the tort system provides an
adversarial court procedure for providing redress for people
injured by negligent care. Negligence is the failure of the
provider to meet an acceptable standard of care owed to the
claimant. Recovery is based on a determination of fault on
the part of the provider. Successful pursuit of a claim usually
necessitates retention of an attorney on a contingent fee basis
(typically calling for a fee of 30 to 50 percent of any recovery).
The litigation process may continue for years after the claim
has been instituted. Damages may be limited to *special damages* such as loss of wages, reduced capacity, and the like.
They may also include noneconomic damages such as payment for pain and suffering. Because noneconomic damages
are highly subjective and often reflect a jury's emotional bias,
they are often excessive in relationship to the special damages
awarded.

Health care providers have been unanimous in their
criticism of the tort system. They say that the system is inef-
fective in discouraging the negligent practitioner and that it
unduly rewards the successful claimant's attorney. They also
maintain that the awards are excessive, especially those for
noneconomic damages; that preparation of the defense is
unduly expensive; and that soaring insurance premium costs
penalize physicians in the higher-risk categories, causing
some to withdraw from the profession or switch to a less
risky premium category. Risk of liability has caused physicians to practice "defensive medicine." This means that they
order all reasonably conceivable laboratory tests for a patient
rather than just those that seem to be clinically appropriate,
so that it will not appear that the doctor has negligently
"missed" something. Over 40 percent of physicians report
ordering more tests in response to increases in liability.[8]

While cost shifting does not directly increase health
care costs, its influence on the way costs are absorbed by the

system has a substantial destabilizing effect on health care payment mechanisms. Cost shifting, in conjunction with direct cost increasing factors, is driving the system into crisis. Cost shifting is the practice of increasing charges to self-pay hospital patients and to indemnity health plans that have no contractual relationship with the hospital that would entitle them to pay less than full hospital charges. For example, Blue Cross, health maintenance organizations (HMOs), and preferred provider organizations (PPOs) contract with hospitals to pay less than hospital charges. To offset this loss and to maintain positive margins (a hospital euphemism for making a profit), an increase is made prospectively to those not entitled to a discount. Additionally, the Medicare prospective payment system frequently reimburses hospitals less than their costs, and Medicaid does so in most states. This means that hospital boards from time to time are called on to approve increases in room charges and fees for ancillary services, like operating rooms, laboratories, and the like, which usually affect only a small percentage of the hospital's patients. For example, if only 25 percent of a hospital's patients are self-pay or their care is reimbursed by an indemnity plan, any increase in charges must be four times the size that would be necessary if there were an "all-payer system" and everyone paid the same amount. Underwriters of indemnity insurance are withdrawing from the market, so that this source of payment is drying up. Escalating prices are converting many uninsured people, who were self-pay, into medically indigent. The cost-shifting process is feeding on itself, getting rapidly worse, and, together with escalating costs and the growing pool of uninsureds, is propelling the health care system into a crisis that can only be resolved by radical reforms.

Many health plans, to improve their economic performance, will not accept members who have chronic health problems, sometimes referred to as preexisting conditions. As writers of these plans become increasingly concerned about the cost of providing benefits, it will become increasingly important that the problem of exclusion from plan enrollment be addressed.

What Proposals for Reform Are Being Considered?

Critics of the health care system are virtually unanimous in their statement of what we should expect to achieve by reform: provide for universal access to services while containing costs. The difficulty is in reaching a national consensus on which of several competing methods we should follow to achieve these ends and, once having agreed on the method, developing a consistent, fully articulated plan to achieve our expectations.

Plans change to conform to change in the circumstances under which they were formulated. The composition of constituencies backing plans changes as the plans change. In health plan support, where one stands often depends on where one sits. It is not likely, for example, that the AFL-CIO, the American College of Physicians, and the National Association of Manufacturers would all find the same health plan ideal.

At this point, it might be useful to discuss a few of the numerous reform plans that have been publicly proposed or introduced in Congress in the form of legislation. The plan that has probably received the most attention has been the program detailed in the *Pepper Commission Report*. Established by the Medicare Catastrophic Coverage Act of 1988 as the U.S. Bipartisan Commission on Comprehensive Health Care, the commission, under the chairmanship of Senator Jay Rockefeller, issued its report in September 1990. To achieve universal health coverage at affordable cost, the commission recommended expansion of employer-based health coverage and the development of a new federal program for nonworkers and the self-employed.

Employers with more than 100 employees would be required to provide health care coverage for employees and their dependents. There would be reforms in the private insurance market, such as the elimination of preexisting conditions as a barrier to coverage. For five years there would be a federal subsidy for employers with fewer than twenty-five workers and an average payroll of less than $18,000 per worker. A new federal health care coverage program would be established that would give employers an alternative to purchasing insurance in the private market. It would be administered through private insurers or the states, subject to federal rules. Price would be set at a specified percentage of the payroll. Medicaid would be replaced with a new program for nonworkers and the self-employed. Nonworkers and the self-employed would receive the same benefits as employees. There would be a minimum standard of coverage for all, which would include primary as well as catastrophic care. Minimum care would include early diagnosis and preventive services. All covered persons, subject to ability to pay, would be expected to pay 20 percent of their premium costs and deductibles, except for preventive services, or $250 per person and $500 per family.

Two health care reform bills have been introduced in the first session of the 102nd Congress. The first to be introduced was sponsored by Senate Majority Leader George J. Mitchell of Maine and Senator Edward M. Kennedy of Massachusetts. This is an employer-based plan providing mandatory coverage for employees. This is a "play or pay" plan that requires all employers to provide basic benefits or pay a 7 percent payroll tax. A presidential commission would be established to set spending limits, and hospital fees would be published. The federal-state Medicaid program would be replaced.

A similar employer based "play or pay" plan was introduced in the house by Rep. Dan Rostenkowski (D-Ill.), chairman of the House Ways and Means Committee. The Rostenkowski bill would require all employers to provide health insurance for their workers or pay a tax of 9 percent. Public coverage would be paid for by a surcharge on individual and corporate income taxes starting at 6 percent in 1993 and increasing to 9 percent in 1996. A national cap on spending would be tied to the rate of growth in the gross national product, adjusted for inflation, plus 4 percent. A national panel would be appointed to negotiate rates with providers, and this rate would apply to all payers.

The National Leadership Commission has proposed a plan that would provide universal access to health care. According to this plan, Medicare would pay for older citizens and employer health plans would cover those who are employed. All others would be covered, either by individual purchases of health insurance or by a fund to be established to provide health care access for them, including those presently covered by Medicaid.

The program would provide for a basic level of health care, the scope of which would be determined by legislation. The plan would be administered by the states, which could provide for benefits in addition to those contained in the national package. The plan calls for cost-sharing provisions such as deductibles and copayments. Employers whose health plans do not provide the mandated basic coverage for all full-time workers would be required to pay a fee for those who were not. All uninsured persons with incomes in excess of 150 percent of the federal poverty level who receive benefits under the plan would be required to pay a fee.

The Enthoven-Kronick proposal is a so-called consumer choice plan. Consumer choice plans are intended to provide incentives to their participants to become cost-conscious health care shoppers. Under this plan, universal health care would be obtained by keeping Medicare and Medicaid in place as well as through employer-based plans. Enthoven-Kronick would add an additional insurer, which would be a sponsor agency in each state. Medicare and Medicaid would continue to cover the people they presently do. Full-time employees and their dependents would receive coverage through their employers, and those without coverage (plus employers who wanted it) would receive coverage through the state agency. Public sponsors would pay and employers would contribute 80 percent of the cost of basic coverage. Employers that had less than twenty-five full-time employees and that arranged coverage through the sponsor agency would not be required to pay more than 8 percent of their payroll for employee health care benefits. Employer contributions exceeding 80 percent would be taxable income to the person benefited, but persons with incomes below 150 percent of the federal poverty level would receive additional federal subsidies without tax penalty. Contributions to the 80 percent subsidy provided by the state sponsor agency would be shared by the state and federal governments, with the federal government paying 50 percent and the state paying 30 percent.

Federal costs would be financed through an 8 percent payroll tax paid by employers on the first half of the social security wage base of wages earned by uncovered part-time employees and by an 8 percent income tax on some part of the adjusted gross income of others, such as early retirees.

The Heritage Foundation also has a consumer choice plan. This plan is designed to encourage Americans to purchase their own health care and health care insurance. Employees would receive tax credits for individual health insurance and for out-of-pocket expenses for health care. Tax credits for out-of-pocket expenses would be larger than those for insurance premiums. This should tend to reduce insurance costs, because it would eliminate many illnesses that the insurer would otherwise have to pay for. If medical insurance should be greater than a specified percentage of family income, there would be cash payments to make up for this. If tax credits should exceed a family's income tax liability, this would be made up for in cash payments. Taxpayers would receive credits for *elective health care payments* for relatives that were not their dependents.

For Medicare recipients, the Part B premium would be eliminated and the Part B deductible would be increased. There would be coinsurance on Part A expenditures. (If you find this confusing, see the discussion of "Reimbursement Under Medicare and Medicaid" in Chapter Nine.) Those covered by Medicare could elect to receive vouchers equal in value to the government's average payment per Medicare recipient. These could be used to pay for health care or for health insurance premiums.

The poor would be covered by the issuance of refundable credits, as would the unemployed. These expenses would be lessened by elective health care payments by relatives under the income tax exception noted above and by insurance that would continue if an employee changed or lost a job.

Several health care plans are modeled on the Canadian system. The federally mandated Canadian system delivers health care on a provincial basis through private sector providers, with all residents of the province included in its coverage. Costs are substantially lower than they are in the United States. In each province, the government acts as the sole provider. Most American versions of the Canadian system would have the states or the federal government acting as the sole provider, with costs paid for by payroll taxes and surtaxes on federal income taxes. Hospitals would be reimbursed at a negotiated rate, and billing would be periodical. Versions of this program have been proposed by Physicians for a National Health Program, the Committee for National Health Insurance, and some of the states.

We will come back to these health plans in Chapter Thirteen when we discuss how trustees of hospitals should respond to different plans and their constituent parts. These plans will affect different hospitals in different ways.

CHAPTER 2

Understanding
the Hospital Setting

The modern hospital is, arguably, the most complex socio-economic organism ever devised. Its organization is unique.

By way of contrast, universities, businesses, and most other organizations in the western world are usually organized as pyramidal-hierarchical structures in which power is concentrated at the top (the chancellor, the president). Power then descends through a widening control/command structure to include, at the bottom level, the most basic unit and lowest control/command rank.[1] The relationship of the organized medical staff of the hospital and of its fee-for-service physicians makes the hospital organization uniquely different. There is no pyramid of power. Each such physician has a direct, one-on-one relationship with the institution.

A qualified physician may be granted staff privileges permitting him or her to utilize hospital facilities within clearly defined limits and subject to the discipline of the clinical organization of the medical staff. In exchange, the physician agrees to abide by the corporate and medical staff bylaws and the rules and regulations of the hospital. In addition, the individual physician may be expected to perform certain services for the hospital, such as teaching medical residents, seeing emergency or charity patients, or supervising the activities of other physicians or allied health care professionals. Collectively, the physicians and allied health care professionals receiving such privileges and acting as the organized medical staff are responsible to the board for all health care delivery within the institution. Although the organized medical staff is a pyramidal-hierarchical structure, this does not alter the relationship of the fee-for-service physicians to the hospital. Fee-for-service physicians are not employees of the hospital and look to their patients for their compensation.

The hospital provides the setting for members of the organized medical staff to practice an ever-expanding number of medical and surgical specialties and subspecialties. These physicians utilize an array of increasingly complex and expensive modalities furnished by the hospital.

The organized medical staff interfaces with an administration headed by a chief executive officer who usually has specialized education and extensive training in the hospital administration field.

Many hospitals have adopted the corporate model for their administrative organization, so that the CEO has the title of president. The senior staff members reporting to him or her are designated vice presidents.[2]

In many cases, the adoption of corporate titles has been accompanied by a change in the manner of managing and governing the institution. Originally organized much like other relatively small charities, hospitals, as they have become large enterprises, have been changing from an *association* form of organization to an *enterprise* or business form. A reexamination of governing board structure, size, and composition has become necessary. Large boards with thirty or more members, selected in many cases to encourage or reward large financial contributions to the hospital, are being replaced by much smaller boards. These board members are now being selected for their individual and collective ability to contribute to the solution of governance problems.[3]

The hospital employs a broad spectrum of medical experts, ranging from physicians and nurses to highly specialized technicians such as kinesiologists, parasitologists, and radiobiologists. It also employs such other skilled and unskilled personnel as may be required to assist in the direct care of its patients and for the administrative management of the institution. It is usually one of the largest employers in its community.

Just What Is a Hospital?

The American Hospital Association defines a hospital as a "health care institution with an organized medical and professional staff and with inpatient beds available around-the-clock, whose primary function is to provide inpatient medical, nursing, and other health-related services to patients for both surgical and nonsurgical conditions, and that usually provides some outpatient, particularly emergency care."[4]

Within this definition, hospitals may be further classified by various characteristics. For example:

> *Voluntary hospitals* are hospitals that are private, not-for-profit, autonomous, self-established, and self-supported.
>
> *Governmental hospitals* are operated by the federal, state, and local governments.
>
> *For-profit hospitals* (sometimes referred to as *investor-owned hospitals*) are usually owned by for-profit corporations to generate a profit for their shareholders.
>
> *General hospitals* treat a wide range of illnesses and injuries.
>
> *Specialty hospitals* may limit treatment to a specific group of patients or illnesses, such as children, mental illnesses, and rehabilitation.
>
> *Teaching hospitals* provide programs in medical, allied health, or nursing education.
>
> *Short-term hospitals* are hospitals whose average length of stay is less than thirty days.
>
> *Long-term hospitals* are hospitals whose patients are not in an acute phase of illness.
>
> *Primary care hospitals* treat the simpler or more common diseases.

Tertiary care hospitals provide highly specialized medical and surgical care for unusual and complex medical and surgical problems.

Community hospitals provide care principally to residents of the community in which the hospital is located.

Regional referral hospitals are ones to which difficult cases are sent for specialized treatment from a wide geographical area.[5]

Ecclesiastical hospitals are hospitals established and operated by a church or religious order.

In total, there are over 6,000 hospitals in the United States. Of these, 3,364 are nongovernment, not-for-profit hospitals. There are 343 federal hospitals, 805 for-profit hospitals, and 1,662 hospitals owned by state and local governments.[6]

The Effect of Socioeconomic Factors on Hospitals

In Chapter One we discussed the current health care crisis. To exercise governance responsibility in an informed manner, trustees must not only understand what the pressures are today but also what pressures have affected the health care system over the past three decades.[7] These pressures include the following:

- Inflation in the health care field that for more than twenty years has substantially exceeded inflation in nearly all other sectors of the economy. The cost of health care in the United States increased from $41.9 billion in 1965 to $750 billion in 1991. This cost is projected to be $1,529.3 billion in the year 2000.[8]
- Increased governmental regulation, principally in an effort to slow the inflationary rate in the health care field and to try to obtain reasonably priced quality health care for Medicare and Medicaid recipients.
- Heavy administrative and auditing costs necessitated by the system.

- Failure of Congress to appropriate, for Medicare purposes, funds to provide reimbursement to hospitals adequate to offset inflationary increases.
- Inadequacy of Medicaid reimbursement in most states.
- Rapid advances in medicine and in medical technology, creating a need for substantial investments of capital by hospitals and demands on them for the provision of new services that these advances have made possible.
- Adoption of a prospective pricing system for Medicare reimbursement (DRGs) that puts hospitals at economic risk with respect to the outcome of treatment as compared with traditional reimbursement systems that are based on hospital charges or costs. DRGs also provide a basis for additional federal controls and standardization of hospitals.
- Broader exposure of hospitals and physicians to tort liability as the result of new case law, the end of the eleemosynary defense, the decline of the locality rule, and the recovery of larger awards by claimants.[9] Doctors are leaving high-risk areas of practice because of staggering malpractice premiums.
- Increased need for health services to care for an aging population.
- The inability of the health care system to attract new nursing and technical personnel to the field in sufficient numbers to meet the system's needs.
- The development of managed care delivery systems such as HMOs and PPOs, whose cost-containment efforts on behalf of their clients tend to reduce hospital admissions and shorten hospital stays.
- The application of antitrust laws to not-for-profit health care providers in the same way that these laws are applied to commercial and industrial enterprises for which they were originally enacted.
- The development of computer-based accounting systems enabling providers to relate the cost of discrete health care services furnished by the institution to the quality of those services.

- Increasing pressure on nonprofit hospitals to establish, on an institution-by-institution basis, the value of social benefits provided by the hospital in exchange for tax exemption and other benefits provided by government.

It is difficult to tell how any given factor, working alone or in combination with others, may have affected hospitals. However, a number of changes have occurred in the hospital field in the last several years that can probably be attributed to the effects of one or more of the preceding conditions. For example, inflation, as previously discussed, has priced more than thirty million uninsured or underinsured Americans out of the health care system.[10] And many hospitals have become highly competitive with one another. Many have established marketing departments and conduct paid advertising campaigns through the media. Hospitals have undergone corporate restructuring, forming for-profit affiliates to try to generate independent streams of revenue from sources other than patient care. The commercialization this has engendered has, among other things, adversely affected the public's image of hospitals and caused federal, state, and local governments to question the appropriateness of hospitals' tax exemptions.

Hospitals have also suffered reductions in their admissions and average length of stay. As a result of technological advances and for cost-containment reasons, many medical conditions that would previously have required hospital admission are now treated on an outpatient basis. Inpatients are more severely ill but are discharged earlier than in the past. As a result of this and overbuilding, many communities have excess hospital beds. To avoid competition with their staff physicians in providing new out-patient services, hospitals are entering into joint ventures with members of their medical staffs. Hospitals are also subsidizing physicians to induce them to join their medical staffs, with a hoped-for resulting increase in hospital admissions. But hospitals are closing, merging, and otherwise trying to survive. And, finally, there are heightened expectations of trustee responsibility and public accountability.

Trends in Hospital Leadership

Fundamental changes in hospital management have occurred over the past two centuries.

Early History: Intrusive Stewardship

In his history of the American hospital system, *The Care of Strangers*,[11] Charles E. Rosenberg notes that in the early nineteenth century, hospitals cared for the urban poor and homeless under intolerably crowded and unsanitary conditions. In those early days when hospitals were small and there were no skilled hospital executives, few trained nurses, and little medical acceptance of the germ theory of disease, trustees exercised a heavy-handed, paternalistic type of stewardship that extended to the smallest operational details of the institutions they served. Because these trustees supported an almost pure charity operation with their own funds, they expected to and did have a dominant and pervasive role in determining how the hospital was run. "Boards of managers," as early governing boards were sometimes called, were managers in a very real sense.

New York Hospital, Rosenberg tells us, had two board committees to exercise oversight functions. The "visiting committee" was entrusted with overseeing admissions.[12] The "inspecting committee" was charged with touring the hospital at least once a week, seeing that "a proper economy" was observed, that the floors were scrubbed and the walls whitewashed, and that the nurses and matron (usually the wife of the superintendent) treated the patients with respect. At Massachusetts General Hospital, the board voted to make its inspection visits unaccompanied by medical staff so that patients and nurses would be encouraged to express possible grievances.

Cavalier notions of the responsibilities of stewardship led some lay boards of the nineteenth century to question certain clinical practices. Sentiment against the consumption of alcoholic beverages impelled some board members to question its therapeutic value. Parsimony brought other lay boards to question the use of expensive leeches to draw blood when lancets had worked well in the past, to limit the number of prescription drugs that could be prescribed by the attending physician, to limit prescriptions to one per patient, and to question the "lavish" use of beef tea and other dietary supplements.[13]

Changes in Board Attitudes

The intrusive activities of lay boards abated as hospitals changed from the almshouses of the eighteenth century to the modern hospitals of the twentieth. These changes have included the following developments:

> The larger size of the institutions as well as their increasing technical complexity, which has resulted from scientific advances. The general public—not just the indigent population—has increasingly come to see hospital inpatient care as an appropriate means of treating injury and disease.[14]
> The establishment of schools of nursing and the development of a corps of skilled nurses.[15]
> The development of increasingly specialized medical staffs, reinforced by trained house officers with responsibilities to the hospital beyond patient care.
> The development of a trained and competent cadre of hospital executives.[16]
> The development of uniform, externally imposed hospital standards by such organizations as the American Hospital Association, the American Medical Association, the American College of Surgeons, and state regulatory agencies.

These and other factors reduced the board's need to intervene in the day-to-day management of the hospital. Increasingly these matters were left to its paid manager.

By the middle of the twentieth century, most boards had

come to regard themselves as merely having responsibility for seeing that their hospitals had sufficient operating funds and an adequate and properly equipped physical plant. The responsibility for seeing that there was a competent medical staff was largely delegated to the staff itself. Providing a competent nursing staff and ensuring compliance with state licensure and practice acts was the responsibility of the administration.

Governing boards had come to believe that they had little or no responsibility for the quality of patient care provided by the medical and nursing staffs within their institutions. Hospital governing boards had largely abdicated their earlier responsibilities.

The Schloendorff Rule. Lack of responsibility of the governing board for the quality of health care delivered within the institution found expression in the *Schloendorff Rule,* based on the decision by Justice Cardoza in *Schloendorff v. Society of New York Hospital* in 1914.[17] The Schloendorff Rule provided that a charitable hospital is not liable for the negligence of its physicians and nurses in the treatment of its patients. The reasoning supporting this rule was that the physicians were independent contractors rather than employees. The hospital, therefore, was not liable for the physicians' actions. The nurses, although employees of the hospital, were under the supervision of a physician in caring for patients. In such circumstances, the nurses were treated as the employees of the physicians rather than the hospital for liability purposes.

The basis for the Schloendorff Rule resulted in a distinction between *medical* and *administrative* functions. When a nurse or other employee of the hospital was performing a medical function under the supervision of a physician, the hospital could not be held liable. But when the nurse was performing an administrative function without physician supervision, the hospital could be held liable.

The application of the Schloendorff Rule distinction between medical and administrative activities produced some seemingly anomalous legal decisions. For example, placing an improperly capped water bottle on a patient's body was held to be administrative, while keeping a hot water bottle on a patient's body too long was held to be medical; transfusing the wrong patient was held to be administrative, while giving the wrong blood to a patient was held to be medical; employing an improperly sterilized needle for a hypodermic injection was administrative, while improperly administering a hypodermic injection was medical; failing to place sideboards on a bed after a nurse decided they were necessary was administrative, while failing to decide that sideboards should be used when the need existed was medical.[18]

The Supreme Court of Illinois put an end to the Schloendorff Rule and its anomalous applications in *Darling v. Charleston Community Memorial Hospital.*[19]

The Darling Case. Dorrence Darling II broke his leg in a football accident on November 5, 1965, and was taken to the emergency room of Charleston Community Memorial Hospital. He was seen there by Dr. John R. Alexander, who was on emergency call that day. Dr. Alexander placed the injured leg in a plaster cast. Not long after the cast was applied, the plaintiff experienced great pain. His toes turned dark and eventually became cold and insensitive. The day after applying the cast, Dr. Alexander notched it around the toes. The following day he cut the cast about three inches up from the foot. On November 8, Dr. Alexander split the cast on each side with a Stryker saw and a stench filled the room. On November 19, the plaintiff was transferred to Barnes Hospital in St. Louis, where the gangrenous leg was eventually amputated.

Darling filed an action charging the hospital with negligence against the hospital. In his complaint, Darling alleged that the hospital was responsible for the negligence of its nurse employees when they failed to monitor and report Darling's condition to the attending physician and, after the physician failed to respond, to report the condition to the hospital administrator. The plaintiff further alleged that the hospital failed to ensure that Dr. Alexander was capable of performing and, in fact, performed his medical services in accordance with standards established by the State Department of Public Health, the Standards for Hospital Accreditation of the American Hospital Association, and the hospital's own bylaws.

In holding that, under the evidence, the jury could have found the defendant hospital liable under either theory of alleged negligence, the court quoted from *Bing v. Thunig* and noted:

> "The conception that the hospital does not undertake to treat the patient, does not undertake to act through its doctors and nurses, but undertakes instead simply to procure them to act upon their own responsibility, no longer reflects the fact. Present-day hospitals, as their manner of operation plainly demonstrates, do far more than furnish facilities for treatment. They regularly employ on a salary basis a large staff of physicians, nurses, and interns [sic], as well as administrative and manual workers, and they charge patients for medical care and treatment, collecting for such services, if necessary, by legal action. Certainly, the person who avails himself of hospital facilities expects that the hospital will attempt to cure him, not that its nurses or other employees will act on their own responsibility."
> (Fuld, J., in *Bing v. Thunig*, (1957) 2 N.Y.2d 656, 163 N.Y. 2d 3, 11, 143 N.E.2d 3, 8.) The Standards for Hospital Accreditation, the state licensing regulations, and the defendant's bylaws demonstrate that the medical profession and other responsible authorities regard it as both desirable and feasible that a hospital assume certain responsibilities for the care of the patient.[20]

Board Responsibility After Darling. The decision in Darling and subsequent cases has established that the hospital board is responsible for the following: establishing a system for credentialing competent physicians, monitoring that system to ensure that staff members maintain an acceptable level of competence, and terminating or limiting the staff privileges of any physician who fails to maintain that level of competence. Under Darling, the institution is not ordinarily responsible for occasional negligence of otherwise competent nonemployee members of the hospital medical staff if its credentialing and monitoring procedures have been correct.

The hospital is directly responsible, however, for the negligence of physicians who are hospital employees acting within the scope of their employment, and for the negligence of its employed nurses. The theory in such cases is that of *respondeat superior*—the master is responsible for the acts of its servants.

In addition to liability under *respondeat superior,* the hospital may also be liable for the negligence of a physician who is not its employee if the public is led to believe that the physician is an employee of the hospital. This is sometimes referred to as *ostensible agency.*

A recent Alaskan court went further, however, and held that where a hospital is mandated by law or by its organic documents (charter or bylaws) to provide a service (such as an emergency room service), such mandate creates a nondelegable duty on the part of the hospital concerning the safety of its patients receiving the service. Consequently, the hospital becomes vicariously liable for the negligence of the physicians providing such service, even if the physicians are independent contractors and there is no ostensible agency.[21]

The End of the Eleemosynary Charitable Defense. Finally, until recent years, some states offered a defense to charitable institutions—the *eleemosynary defense.* When sued for negligence, charitable institutions could raise their charitable nature as an absolute defense against any claims for tort liability. The theory was that the assets of an eleemosynary institution were held in trust for the accomplishment of its charitable purposes and could not be diverted to provide reparations for a person injured by the institution's negligence. Often criticized, the eleemosynary defense was rejected during the 1950s and 1960s by nearly all states.

CHAPTER 3

The Nature
of the Hospital Board

The law imposes the legal, moral, and ethical responsibility for the operation of the hospital on a board that is usually composed largely, if not entirely, of lay members. Until joining the hospital board, most of these volunteers have not had even the slightest experience in the health care field other than as recipients of care. One writer noted:

> With more than $72 billion worth of assets in the health care industry, and an annual rate of spending currently in excess of $100 billion a year [This was written in 1982. In 1991, the latter figure had risen to $750 billion a year.] . . . it is somewhat shocking to realize that the ultimate responsibility for spending and investing these billions rests with part-time, unpaid volunteer workers called hospital trustees.
>
> In addition to financial responsibility, hospital trustees have legal responsibility for the quality and appropriateness of care for some 36 million people admitted to hospitals each year as inpatients. They also are responsible for ambulatory care for more than a quarter of a billion outpatient visitors each year to emergency depart-

ments, outpatient clinics, diagnostic centers, and
therapy departments.

Daily hospital operations are run by administrators and the medical staff determines and sup-
plies the medical treatment of patients. But it is
the hospital governing board—the trustees—that
evaluates management plans and performance
and provides or denies the funding for medical
equipment, staff facilities, investment, and capital
assets.[1]

One of the strengths of our voluntary hospitals is their
unique system of governance. Just as war is too important to
be left to the generals, the governance of our hospitals is
too important to be left to the hospital management and
physicians.

Board Leadership Qualities

Board leadership qualities encompass a wide range of attributes and areas of expertise.

Basic Traits

A discussion of board leadership qualities might well begin
with a list of some of the basic traits all board members
should ideally possess. Cyril Houle makes the following suggestions: "Perhaps the most frequently mentioned [leadership
traits] are commitment to the importance of the service or
function with which the board is to be concerned, a respected
position in the community, intelligence, courage, capacity
for personal growth, the ability to influence public opinion
among significant sectors of the community, willingness to
serve, and readiness to work with others."[2]

Board leadership usually manifests itself through committee activity. A board member develops expertise in one of
the fields a committee deals with. Colleagues on the board
tend increasingly to defer in this area to that member's exper-

tise, and ultimately this is reflected in an assignment as committee chair. The committee chair should meet regularly with the senior management representative who staffs the committee and thus has further opportunities to develop expertise through regular consultation with a professional in the field.

Progress toward the position of board chair usually occurs through the leadership of several committees. The person ultimately selected to act as board chair will be someone who has a compelling interest in the hospital and the ability to devote substantial amounts of time to hospital matters on a daily basis.

The effective chair must have good people skills, be able to work closely with the board and its individual members, the CEO, and others who are part of the hospital's "family"—medical staff, facility users, and contributors. This person must also have a detailed knowledge of the hospital's operations as well as of what is going on in health care in the community and across the country. In addition, the chair must have the continued unwavering support of the board and the respect of the community.

Negative Leadership Traits

Perhaps, as a study in contrasts, it would be worthwhile to discuss some of the characteristics that tend to detract from an otherwise qualified person's ability to be an effective board leader. Such negative qualities are not always easy to identify. One example of false board leadership is found in the *expediter,* a person who has more important things to do and wants to see the meeting adjourned as quickly as possible so that he can get on to his next meeting. Many years ago, for example, before cost containment became such an acute and painful issue for hospitals, this often occurred whenever the introduction of a new health program was discussed. Once it had been established to the satisfaction of the board that the program was medically desirable, debate on the economic aspects of the program would frequently be foreclosed by an expediter asking, "Is this reimbursable?" The implication was clear that if the new program was reimbursable, there was no useful purpose to be served by debating whether or not the program was economically sound. Someone else would have to pay the expenses; let someone else worry about the cost. Once the board was satisfied that the program was medically desirable and that the cost would be reimbursed by a third-party payer, the adoption of the program was virtually assured. This type of "leadership," while expediting agenda business at board meetings, annually added cost to health care delivery by tens by millions of dollars. Today, we have a better understanding of fiscal responsibility. When a new program is proposed, with or without certificate of need, fiscal soundness is given at least equal time with medical desirability.

We must continue to look for leadership from trustees who will be willing to engage in in-depth discussions of agenda issues.

I identify many negative leadership traits with the *divine right of governance* syndrome, an affliction that besets some trustees who have sat on too many charitable boards without sufficient qualifying experience in the real world and whose succession to hospital leadership may have resulted more from family prominence than from distinguished community service.

One such negative trait would be a need to dominate. Leadership and domination are quite different. A chair who seeks to dominate his CEO or fellow board members is weakening rather than strengthening the institution. The need is for a chair whose leadership instincts will be to strengthen the CEO and other members of the board in order to provide a strong partnership in support of the institution. It is a synergistic relationship among these leaders that will serve to accomplish the institution's purposes.

A second deterrent to leadership, commonly found in divine righters, is a tendency to "shoot from the hip," without adequate thought or consultation. Very few problems that require resolution by the board's leadership have only a single facet. Such problems are usually multiform and require contemplation and discussion. The solution of one aspect of a problem can frequently create two more problems to take the first one's place. A simplistic solution to a problem involving the retention of the chief executive officer, for example, may lead to embarrassment and great expense in terminating the CEO if his or her continuance in office is later thought by the board to no longer be in the institution's best interests.

A third deterrent to board leadership is the inability of some divine righters to perceive when they have gone beyond the bounds of their own personal abilities in decision making and should defer to someone with special experience or training. Such leaders will take positions on sophisticated legal, accounting, financial, and other matters with respect to which they have no experience or training and will fail to obtain or will ignore the advice of those who do. Their positions are often based on an imperfectly remembered or understood article they have read in a periodical or a conversation they have had with someone thought to be knowledgeable in the field. This is sometimes all the information these individuals feel they need to consider before subjecting their institutions to potential antitrust or tort liability, the sanctions of a credentialing organization, or a default under the covenants of its mortgage indenture.

Another type of problem that relates to the divine right syndrome is an atavistic resistance to change, which may, for example, lead to an insistence that any new problem be accorded the same solution as a superficially similar problem that occurred years earlier, even though the law and accounting rules have changed in the interim and the controlling facts, as seen by other board members, may appear to be quite different. For the divine righter, change is to be avoided and can be avoided even if only by failing to recognize it.

Role of the Chair

Returning to the positive side, let us assume that Pillhaven Hospital has found a person with adequate leadership skills to assume the chair of that institution. What activities should that person be expected to perform individually in exercising the leadership function, in addition to acting in concert with other members of the governing board? We have previously noted that boards act collectively, with certain exceptions. Exercise of the leadership role by the chair is one of those exceptions.

The first responsibility of the chair, acting individually, is to serve for the CEO as the embodiment of the board. In its relationship with the CEO, the board must speak with one voice, and that voice is that of the chair. The chair and the CEO must forge a partnership that will enable the CEO to carry out executive responsibilities in a manner satisfactory to the board and in the best interests of the institution. There must be an atmosphere of mutual trust and confidence. It is easier to define the separate roles of the CEO and the chair than it is to draw a line between them as they develop on a day-to-day basis. If the partnership is a close one, some overlap is bound to exist. This should be a basis for cooperation rather than controversy. Often, the success or failure of the institution will parallel the success or failure of the relationship between the chair and the CEO.

By its very nature, the chair's responsibility in this regard is not delegable.

Other areas in which the chair acts as an individual on behalf of the board include interpreting the institution's role in health care to the community and its leadership, ensuring that the hospital's capital needs are met, and acting as an advocate for the institution with representatives of the local, state, and national governments. These responsibilities are delegable and are shared on a mutually agreeable basis with the CEO and the management team.

Board Role Versus Management Role

Later, we will discuss the concept that the governing board is the proxy for the community served by the hospital. To have any meaning, this concept must be based on the assumption that the societal interest of the community is broader than that of the institution itself and that it is this broader interest that is served by the board. The CEO, on the other hand, is employed by the board to serve the narrower, institutional interests of the hospital. This can, at least theoretically, be the basis for a divergence of perspective between the board and its CEO. For example, at a time when reimbursement and other income is inadequate to meet the hospital's economic needs, to what extent should these needs be met from the hospital's previously accumulated surpluses, when to do so may prejudice future hospital operations? The resolution of this problem may result in the board and the CEO, quite properly, coming down on different sides of the issue. Perhaps a clearer situation where institutional and societal interests may diverge is where an institution considers offering a new medical service that is already being offered by another hospital serving the community. The result, if the new program is successful, will be a strengthening of the institution proposing to offer the new service and a weakening of the institution already offering it. This will impact negatively on the community. What standard should be applied by the governing board proposing to adopt the new service? Obviously, the public interest should prevail over that of the individual institution. In effect, the governing board should vote against the putative interest of its hospital.

The Board as Proxy for the Community

The central tenet of nonprofit hospital governance is that the governing board collectively acts as a proxy for the community the hospital serves. Although the members of the board may not be physicians or hospital managers, they should bring to the hospital's affairs not only their collective wisdom and experience but also a detachment and balanced judgment that, in sum, fully and fairly reflects the community's expectations for the institution.

The weakness in this system is that many trustees fail to develop enough knowledge of the hospital and of the responsibilities of a trustee to be able to contribute effectively to the decisions of the board and the recommendations of its committees. An uninformed or indifferent board simply is not up to the complicated task of establishing and auditing hospital policy in an era of increasing competition and diminishing resources.

Worse, an uninformed or indifferent board could cause a role reversal between management and the governing board. When this happens, the board ceases to function in its ordained role. By default, management assumes the responsibilities of governance and the board is advised by management as to the institution's policies and plans. Critics of the hospital organizational structure have concluded that to prevent such a role reversal from taking place, a statutory framework should be developed to ensure that the direction of hospital managerial control rests squarely with the governing body.[3]

To adequately discharge its responsibility to the community, every hospital board should have at least a small core of knowledgeable and dedicated trustees who have, in essence, made hospital board membership a second career.

Management Distinguished

The board does not manage the hospital. Instead, the hospital is managed by professional managers under a CEO who is selected by and who reports to the board. The day-to-day activities that take place within the hospital other than the actual delivery of medical care by physicians and paramedical personnel are the responsibility of the CEO.

The board monitors the execution of policy by the hospital's management. It acts as an enlightened "backseat driver."

Policy and Oversight

The board establishes policy. It adopts a *mission statement*, which briefly summarizes the hospital's role in the community. The board determines the services to be provided by the hospital now and in the future, and how the assets of the hospital are to be allocated among those services and with respect to the hospital's plant and equipment. The board exercises oversight responsibility as to the credentialing of physicians and other health care professionals and, through the organized medical staff, monitors the discharge of their professional responsibilities. The board is responsible for the quality of care delivered in the institution. The board ensures that the hospital serves the needs of the community as they are perceived by the board and reflected in the hospital's mission statement.

Boards Act Collectively: Exceptions

Governing boards, with some exceptions, act collectively. It is to the collective wisdom of the board, not to that of any individual member, that the community has entrusted the hospital's governance. The community is entitled to the benefit of the board's collective wisdom. The exceptions to this are situations in which the board delegates the power to act on a specific matter to particular board members or to a standing or ad hoc committee.

The chair, to exercise the leadership function, must act independently of the board, particularly in relation to the CEO. In a well-run hospital, the chair and CEO should be a smooth-running, well-integrated team working in harmony with each other so that the not-always-distinct division between governance and management becomes invisible.

The danger in such a close working relationship between the board chair and CEO is that the two of them together may tend to make decisions that should be reserved for the full board and thus transform what should be a democratic process into an autocratic one.

Another exception to the rule that the board should act collectively is when the board has an executive committee, which, under the bylaws, may exercise the power of the full board when the board is not in session.

Board Composition

The mechanics of selecting hospital board members varies from institution to institution. In a not-for-profit hospital, the board may be self-perpetuating and elect its own members, or, if it is a membership model, the members elect the board. In a restructured hospital setting, the parent corporation usually names the hospital's board. Whatever the mechanics, the following suggestions should be appropriate.

Suggested Criteria for Board Selection

First of all, the present trend is away from boards composed, as they often were in the past, on the basis of encouraging or rewarding substantial contributors. These boards tended to be large and composed of people of prominence in the community without regard for the individual qualities, experiences, and abilities they brought to the board table. As the ability of hospitals to be financially self-sustaining and to generate capital through borrowings has increased with the advent of health insurance and Medicare, financial reliance on affluent or influential board members has diminished. Today, hospitals are downsizing boards and bringing a spectrum of varied talents and experience to their governance. Therefore, the focus now is on increasing the diversity of board members, so as to make the hospital board greater than the sum of its parts.

Because the board ordinarily acts collectively, an effort should be made to see that it is composed of a cross section of community leadership. As Frederick H. Kerr notes, "Trustees should be chosen for their ability to function as governors and policy makers. They must be people who can perceive the role of governance clearly, avoid conflicts of interest (including not serving as a director or employee of a competing organization), conceptualize policy questions, perceive health services from a community standpoint, understand professionalism, appreciate management considerations, en-

courage forward looking strategies, prepare for and attend
meetings regularly, and have a genuine interest in the health
needs of the population served."[4]

John A. Witt, an author and hospital consultant, suggests ten criteria for board selection:

- Experience—Participation on other voluntary boards
- Achievement—Business or professional success
- Skills—Talents that will broaden the capabilities of the board player
- Teamwork—The ability to work in harmony with other board members
- Affluence—If all other criteria are satisfied
- Positive Associations—Good personal or family member experience with the hospital
- Personal Qualities—A good listener, intelligent, and known to be of high moral and ethical standards
- Objectivity—Someone representing no one group in particular
- Commitment—Readiness to remain a member over the long haul
- Receptivity to Training—Willingness to develop and improve trustee skills[5]

Witt's suggestions relate to the selection of what
might be described as a *community representative* board.

In its publication *Governance Issue Briefings*, the Illinois Hospital Association suggests a method of selecting
what may be called an *enterprise board*, one that targets
board members with differing complementary skills:

- Assess the attributes of the present board, including occupation, years of service, and other board memberships.
- Identify the current board's strengths and weaknesses. Are

certain professions overrepresented or different skills needed?

- Determine the needed mix of skills for the future using the strategic plan as the guide. For example, recruitment of a marketing professional with knowledge of women's issues may be appropriate if increasing the market share of the recently built women's health center is a priority. The intent is not to supplant management's role in this area but to complement it.

- Prepare job descriptions for officers, committee chairmen, and board members, outlining the overall roles and responsibilities for these positions to assist such persons in understanding what is expected of them and for use as a recruitment tool.

- Use a subcommittee for accomplishing the previous four tasks. Then the entire board should be presented with the information and the subcommittee's recommendations for types of nominees. All board members should be requested to suggest nominees. An effective way to get input is to distribute a form to board members requesting suggestions.

- Recruit potential nominees selected by the full board. The recruiters should be small in number and include the chief executive and the committee members who have the best relationship with the nominees. A potential nominee should be given a thorough explanation of the roles, responsibilities, and expectations of board members. Too often the explanation of the duties that accompany the honor of being a trustee is inadequate. Then, following appointment, other board members are disappointed by the new member's poor attendance at meetings or hospital functions. Small boards, in particular, suffer when there are non-contributing members. Do not beg a candidate. People who cannot make the required commitment when asked should still be kept in mind for the future through a catalog or other means of listing prospective members.[6]

Criticism of Board Composition

Despite the availability of criteria for developing well-balanced and effective board organizations, hospital boards tend to follow certain patterns in selecting members and, when the board is self-perpetuating, they often select as successors people who are like themselves.

Surveys have shown that hospital trustees are mostly between the ages of forty and sixty-five, Caucasian, male, Protestant, with baccalaureate degrees and some graduate training. They are largely executives, managers, bankers, attorneys, and teachers. They earn substantial incomes.[7]

Critics of the health care system have pointed out the narrowly elitist structure of many hospital boards and have suggested that the hospital's community would be better served if there were more consumers, women, and minorities represented on hospital boards and if board members were residents of the community where the hospital is located.

One state, in fact, passed legislation to ensure that voluntary hospital boards in that state would be more representative of the community as a whole. In 1983, the West Virginia legislature enacted what is now Section 16-5B-6(a) of the West Virginia Code.[8] This statute requires that at least 40 percent of the board of directors of all nonprofit and local government hospitals in West Virginia be composed of an equal proportion of "consumer representatives" from four categories: small business, organized labor, elderly persons, and persons whose income is less than the national median income. The act further requires that serious consideration be made to selecting women, minorities, and disabled persons. The constitutionality of this act has been sustained by the U.S. District Court for the Northern District of West Virginia,[9] and this decision has been confirmed by the Fourth Circuit Court of Appeals.[10]

While the West Virginia statute does have the advantage of getting concerned people involved in hospital policy, it has numerous objectionable aspects. Are the consumer representatives drawn from the four mandated categories going to represent all users of the hospital's services or are they going to tend to represent their own particular concerns? Are the consumer representatives going to be able to work harmoniously with the other board members who have been, presumably, chosen from the categories traditionally represented on hospital boards? Does the addition of these consumer representatives to the board strengthen or weaken the institution? Has this type of board reform improved the delivery of health care in West Virginia?

Leslie Levy of the Harvard Business School views board reform with caution.[11] She believes that structural reform without other changes will not improve board effectiveness. What we need, she says, is not merely capable individuals composing the board, but, more important, a capable group. The board must be able to function as a working entity. It must develop the capability to collectively discuss the issues brought before it. It must develop the knowledge, attitude, and skills necessary to effectively address the institution's problems.

Downsizing the Board

Community representative boards tend to become too large to permit all members to participate in the governance function. If the board wishes to change to an enterprise form of board, it may wish to reduce its size. Downsizing an existing board whose members have demonstrated loyalty to the institution over the years, but where sheer size impedes the governance process, is problematical. Abruptly dropping prominent community leaders from the board could have adverse consequences for the institution's relationship with the community. In a hospital organized as a membership corporation, however, some board members might not only be willing to become members instead of trustees but might welcome this opportunity. The burden of being a member—that is, attending the annual election of board members and approving changes in the corporation's organic structure, such as charter and bylaw amendments—is much less than that of board membership. However, members retain a personal identification with the institution and can be expected to show continued support. In an institution with a self-perpetuating board, consideration might be given to a charter amendment (if state law permits) to convert to a membership corporation. The members could then be recruited from the board, reducing it to a workable size. Adopting a designation for the members such as *board of corporators, board of overseers,* or *board of visitors* and giving them some additional identification with the institution might confer added prestige and make the change from trustee to member more attractive.

Length of Term

How long should a trustee serve? Most trustees are elected to serve for one-, two-, or three-year terms of office. Usually when the term is for two or three years, the trustees are elected by classes, with one-half or one-third of the board members being elected in each year.

Some hospitals have bylaw provisions that require board members to be rotated off the board after they have served a specified number of years or terms on the board. This rotation has certain advantages. It brings more members of the public with fresh ideas into board positions and tends to reduce the possibility of a small clique getting control of the institution. On the other hand, a hospital is such a complex organization that it takes years for a new trustee to gain enough experience to be able to make a contribution to its governance. A policy of automatically rotating trustees off the board will systematically deprive the institution of its most experienced trustees. The hospital might be better off if there were no such bylaw provision and if the nominating committee simply selectively failed to renominate those board members who were not making satisfactory contributions to the hospital's governance and indefinitely retained those who were.

Aside from a record of attendance at board meetings, it is difficult to find an objective basis for evaluating the contribution of an individual board member. Unfortunately, value judgments as to questions asked or suggestions made during meetings will tend to be subjective. Nevertheless, at the time they are called on to prepare a slate of nominees, nominating committees should have a sense of those who have made a real contribution to the institution that merits their retention on the board, and those who have not.

Where there is no automatic rotation off the board, consideration should be given to automatic rotation of board memberships and chair assignments to avoid stagnation of leadership.

In an era when the tenure of senior management is painfully brief, the board must act as the corporate memory. Let us not shorten that memory unnecessarily.

CHAPTER 4

Voluntarism and the Nonprofit Corporation

Except for small physician-owned hospitals in the South and West, there were virtually no for-profit general hospitals in this country before the adoption of Medicare in 1965. It was the adoption of Medicare and the development of the third-party-payer system of reimbursing hospitals for their patient services that enabled for-profit hospitals to obtain capital, construct or acquire hospital facilities, and operate those facilities in multihospital chains. These often have returned handsome profits to their shareholders and, in many cases, have provided their founders with substantial fortunes.

Voluntarism Today

By way of contrast, the not-for-profit hospitals continue the tradition of voluntarism. No individuals benefit financially from the success of their operations. In fact, if their operations result in private inurement to an individual, the requirements of the Internal Revenue Code for tax exemption are violated. The institution's exempt status under federal tax law could be terminated.

Peter F. Drucker points out what an enormous effect the nonprofit sector has on America today: "Few people are aware that the nonprofit sector is by far America's largest employer. Every other adult—a total of 80 million plus people—works as a volunteer, giving on average nearly five hours each week to one or several nonprofit organizations. This is equal to 10 million full time jobs. Were volunteers paid their wages, even at minimum rate, this would amount to some $150 billion, or 5% of GNP."[1] The governing boards of not-for-profit hospitals have traditionally served without compensation, as have members of numerous hospital auxiliaries and individual volunteers who have supported these institutions. All have served to enhance American traditions of altruism and community service.

Most volunteer trustees of nonprofit hospitals have derived a sense of satisfaction from their activities as board members and have been disinclined to engage in critical examinations of the governance mechanism. Nevertheless, such critical examinations have been made, with the examiners in some cases giving the nonprofit corporation poor marks.

The Nonprofit Corporation

A trustee of a not-for-profit corporation should understand the corporate difference between this type of institution and a hospital operated as a for-profit business venture.

Superficially, for-profit and not-for-profit corporations have certain similarities. Each provides for the formation, management, and governance of an artificial corporate entity. Each has charter documents issued by the state that set forth, among other things, its purposes, the length of its existence, the location of its initial registered office, and the names and addresses of its initial board of directors. Additionally, a for-profit corporation's charter will make provision for its capitalization and for the relative rights and preferences of its security holders.

Many state nonprofit corporation statutes permit two alternate corporate governance structures. The first provides for both members and directors. In this configuration, members are analogous to shareholders in the for-profit sector. The members elect the directors and usually must approve major corporate changes, such as amendments to the corporate charter or bylaws.

The other type of permissible governance mechanism is one in which there are no members. The directors are a self-perpetuating group that reelects itself and has no other group such as members from which it must obtain approval for major corporate changes (although in a restructured hospital it may be necessary to secure approval for such changes from the corporate parent).

The self-perpetuating board form of structure has been adopted frequently by hospitals in recent years because it provides a streamlined form that simplifies the mechanics of ensuring continuity of governance and effecting corporate change. Critics point out that the restraint provided by the board having to obtain approvals from the members provides a protection for the public against a board that may not always be acting in the public interest.

The analogy between the shareholders of a for-profit corporation and the members of a nonprofit corporation is not, however, a perfect one. The shareholders of a for-profit corporation clearly have the economic interest of the corporation as their prime consideration. The members of a nonprofit corporation have no such polestar to inform their judgment. In a nonprofit corporation with members, it is possible for individuals with a partisan agenda to gain control of the membership and, through the members' control of the governing board, cause the corporation's activities to be influenced by that partisan interest. Such members could, for example, eliminate from board membership anyone who failed to filter board decisions through any number of biases unrelated to relevant governance concerns (for example, pro-life or pro-choice positions). Since the action of the members in controlling board membership is indirect, it is difficult to obtain effective judicial review of the members' actions. The actions of the governing board, however, are more amenable to judicial scrutiny because it acts directly.

Both for-profit and not-for-profit corporations adopt bylaws that provide for the corporation's governance and management as permitted by the state corporation laws and within any limitations set forth in the charter. But the purpose of a for-profit corporation is to make money for the security holders for whom it is operated, to pay dividends, and to give its shareholders an opportunity for capital appreciation. The purpose of a not-for-profit corporation is to provide services to the public, to which it is ultimately accountable.

The state acts as *parens patriae* or "parent of the country" with respect to the proper application of assets held for charitable purposes, including those held by not-for-profit corporations. The state's powers as *parens patriae* are exercised by the state attorney general.

Federal Income Tax Exemption

For the voluntary hospital organized as a not-for-profit corporation, it is important to obtain and maintain exemption from federal income taxation. The basis for this exemption is Section 501(c)(3) of the Internal Revenue Code of 1986.[2] This section, in relevant part, exempts corporations and any community chest, fund, or organization organized and operated exclusively for religious, charitable, literary, or educational purposes, provided that no part of its net earnings inure to the benefit of any private shareholder or individual, that no substantial part of its activities is carrying on propaganda or attempting to influence legislation, and that it does not participate in or intervene in any political campaign on behalf of a candidate for public office.

Even though it believes itself to be exempt, a voluntary hospital must file an application for exemption with the Internal Revenue Service on Form 1023.

Section 501(c)(3) of the Internal Revenue Code does not have a specific provision exempting hospitals. If hospitals are going to qualify for exemption, they must establish that they are "charitable" within the meaning of the tax code. Prior to 1969, the Internal Revenue Service required that hospitals, to be held to be charitable, had to be operated to the extent of their financial ability for those not able to pay for the services rendered and not exclusively for those who were able and expected to pay.[3]

In 1969, the Internal Revenue Service issued Revenue Ruling 69-545, which altered its position and no longer required hospitals to render free care to the poor in order to be classified as charitable.[4] In this ruling, the Internal Revenue Service recognized health care as a charitable purpose without regard for relief of the poor. To be exempt under the ruling, a hospital must promote the health of a class of persons broad enough to benefit the entire community it serves and must be operated to serve a public rather than a private interest. The emergency room must be open to all in need of emergency care (even if they cannot pay), and the hospital itself must be open to all who have the ability to pay. The fact that the hospital's receipts may exceed its expenses does not disqualify it from exemption.

Although Rev. Rul. 69-545 is still in effect, there is likely to be a change in the requirements for exemption from federal income taxation. Representative Brian Donnelly (D-Mass.) has introduced a bill that would require all hospitals, as a condition of tax exemption, to maintain open emergency rooms and to annually provide charity care equivalent to 5 percent of their gross revenues. Although Donnelly's bill has received little support during the first session of the 102nd Congress, congressional sentiment seems to be moving away from support for an exemption such as that provided for in Rev. Rul. 69-545 and toward an exemption requiring substantial provision of uncompensated care.

It should be noted that obtaining a ruling as to tax exemption (frequently referred to as the *determination letter*) does not exempt the institution from payment of taxes on income derived from activities not related to its tax exempt purposes, that is, *unrelated business income*.[5]

Trustees should also know that activities that would be exempt if performed by their institution acting alone may be taxable if performed in conjunction with one or more other exempt hospitals unless the activity is specifically referred to in Section 501(e) of the code.[6] Central laundries operated by two or more hospitals to take care of their own laundry needs, for example, are not listed in Section 501(e), and their activities are taxable. Even if the activity is listed in Section 501(e), the exemption provided by that section is not the equivalent of exemption provided by Section 501(c)(3). An organization exempt under Section 501(e) may not accumulate earnings to enhance its ability to carry out its charitable purposes but must be organized as a cooperative and annually pay out its net earnings to its patrons on the basis of services performed for them.[7]

State laws relating to exemption of hospital properties from *ad valorem* real estate taxes vary from state to state and within a given state. The criteria for exempting hospital property from real estate taxes may differ from those relating to the application of state sales and use taxes or corporate net income taxes. The basis for the exemption is the charitable nature of the hospital.

Recently, the taxing bodies imposing state and local real estate taxes in several states have challenged the exempt status of hospitals within their jurisdictions. Many of these taxing bodies had observed that the hospitals, with the benefit of payments from health insurance and Medicare, were providing much less free care than they had when they were founded and received their tax exemptions. Some of the taxing bodies also noted that many restructured hospitals in their jurisdictions appeared to have departed from their primary roles of providing health care, irrespective of the patient's ability to pay. Instead, they appeared to be primarily concerned with the promotion of various business activities, often in competition with local businesses. For example, in *School District of the City of Erie v. The Hamot Medical Center* (Erie County, Pennsylvania, No. 138-A-1989), in sustaining the revocation of real estate tax exemption for a large tertiary care hospital, the court found that the hospital's primary purpose was no longer charitable. The hospital had restructured, forming twenty corporations, including some for-profit corporations, that were engaged in constructing office buildings, developing real estate, and operating a marina, a health club, a telephone answering service, and a retirement home. It had transferred $25 million of the surplus it had made in the previous eight years to its affiliates.

In reaching its conclusion that Hamot Medical Center did not meet the state law requirements for exemption from real estate taxation, the court looked at the totality of the circumstances of Hamot's operations. In addition to the contributions of uncompensated care, the judge gave consideration to Hamot's contributions to community benefit programs, health education, and medical research. Rather than resorting to a formulaic analysis of the amount of uncompensated care provided by Hamot, the judge considered whether the hospital made a bona fide effort to serve those who could not afford to pay. A narrower test is one based on a mathematical formula for determining how much free care should be provided by a hospital as a condition of real estate tax exemption. But this appears to be too narrow a test for determining tax exemption today. If hospitals are not to receive automatic tax exemption, and it seems that they are not, the test for exempt status should be an examination of the totality of circumstances, as was done in the Hamot case. The court should look to see what community service is rendered by the hospital for which it is not compensated or is inadequately compensated. This would include the provision of free care. The value of these community benefits would then be balanced against the value to the institution of exemption from taxation.

In Vermont, to qualify for exempt status, it is merely necessary for the hospital to make health care available to all who need it, irrespective of ability to pay. No formulaic amount of free care is required.[8] Utah, on the other hand, requires a certain level of free care to support real estate tax exemption.[9]

Some hospitals whose real estate tax exemption has been questioned have felt concerned that as good citizens they should, without giving up their tax exemption, make some contribution to the cost of municipal services provided to them, such as fire and police protection. These hospitals have accomplished this by negotiating agreements to make payments in lieu of taxes. These are usually for more than one year and are usually conditioned on the taxing bodies agreeing not to raise the exemption issue while the payments are being made.

Governing boards should be sure that they are currently informed as to the status of their income tax and real estate exemptions. Trustees should try to influence tax legislation constructively to the extent they are able. They should have counsel advise them of any action on the part of local taxing bodies to strip them of their real estate tax exemption and should ensure that the hospital is in a position to justify its claim to exempt status on the basis of benefits provided to the community, including free care. The trustees should be given the opportunity to consider, if their real estate exemption is threatened, whether they wish to enter into an agreement to make payments in lieu of taxes, either as a matter of conscience or to avoid the expenses and hazards of litigation. Entering into such an agreement without a threat to exemption, however, might subject the governing board to a claim that it had wasted a corporate asset.

Criticisms of the Nonprofit Corporation

Robert Charles Clark, writing in the *Harvard Law Review* in 1980, found much to criticize about nonprofit corporations owning and operating hospitals. The abstract appearing at the beginning of his article sums it up concisely:

> Nonprofit hospitals currently enjoy favored legal status. . . . Professor Clark . . . begins by identifying problems in the health care industry and then explores the relationship between nonprofit hospitals and these problems. He finds that the evidence does not persuasively establish that nonprofit hospitals serve as fiduciaries rather than exploiters and that nonprofits engage in much

involuntary cross-subsidization of medical services. He concludes that the legal favoritism for
the nonprofit form is based not on sound reasoning and hard data but on intuition. Professor
Clark proposes that the legal rules affecting nonprofit hospitals reflect this reality by treating
both nonprofits and for-profits neutrally by controlling cross-subsidization, and by strengthening
consumer information about and control over
health care decision making.[10]

Robin Dimieri and Stephen Weiner, in an article in
the *Vanderbilt Law Review,* conclude that for nonprofit hospitals to have a governance structure adequate to protect the
public interest in a competitive system, it would be necessary
to enact legislation making the responsibility of nonprofit
corporate members more analogous to that of for-profit corporate shareholders. They also suggest that the corporate
structure that provides for a self-perpetuating governing
board without corporate members is inadequate for purposes
of hospital governance.[11]

It should be noted that Clark's article and that of
Dimieri and Weiner assume that one of the objectives of governance is to facilitate public participation in or control of
the governance process. Many professionals in the hospital
field, however, believe strongly that hospital policy development is not facilitated by debating it at a New England town
meeting type of forum. If this criticism is accepted, the two
articles, considered from this viewpoint, may be somewhat
flawed.

Writing in the *Harvard Business Review,* Regina E.
Herzlinger and William S. Krasker maintain that although
nonprofit hospitals receive more social subsidies than for-
profits, they do not achieve better results for society. They are
not more accessible to those unable to pay and they are as
expensive as the for-profit hospitals. The nonprofits replace
plant and equipment more slowly than the for-profits. For-
profits require little societal investment. They are more effi-

cient than nonprofits and offer as broad a range of services, including services to the medically indigent.[12]

Although Herzlinger and Krasker's article has also been criticized, the three articles taken together indicate that some highly regarded academics at prestigious institutions do not regard the nonprofit corporation as the ideal instrument for health service delivery. They question whether the nonprofit hospitals deserve the social subsidies they receive. In view of these searching criticisms and given public efforts to eliminate hospital exemptions from *ad valorem* real estate and other taxes, hospital boards should carefully examine their organizational structures to make sure that they can convince the public of their social value and that they merit their continued preferred status.

CHAPTER 5

Recruiting
and Retaining the CEO

Selection and retention of the right CEO are extremely important to the success of any hospital. The board should take great care in both these areas.

Recruiting the CEO

Recruiting a CEO is a task most hospital trustees perform at least once during their board tenure. Choosing the right person to fill this position is of paramount importance to the institution, because the CEO will have more influence on the operation and success of the hospital than the board will. While a certain amount of subjectivity will enter the process (every hospital is different, and the right person for one institution may not be the right person for another), there are certain common characteristics that should be sought in any candidate.

Candidates should be people of good character who will fairly represent the institution in and to the community. They should be dedicated to the institution and to its goals. They should be able to deal diplomatically, but effectively, with members of the medical staff and the board. They should be capable of dealing objectively with complex matters and of finding acceptable solutions to problems that may initially appear to be intractable. They should be leaders who instill a sense of loyalty in subordinates and a sense of confidence in members of the board and medical staff. They should have a particular facility in dealing with financial and accounting matters. They should be patient and respectful of the points of view of others.

Most candidates will have an undergraduate or graduate degree in hospital administration, perhaps both, and will probably have served either as CEO of a small hospital or as a senior manager at a comparable hospital. Alternatively, the candidate may already be employed by the hospital as a member of senior management and have attained a favorable reputation among peers and members of the board.

In evaluating an executive's previous experience in a for-profit setting, the board of a nonprofit hospital should be aware that the executive may be inexperienced in dealing with nonsalaried physicians and almost certainly will be without experience in fundraising and corporate development. Experience in the for-profit area should, however, have produced an executive with a strong orientation toward bottom-line results, a very valuable trait in today's environment.

Candidates should have personality traits that will enhance their ability to work with members of the governing board. Since hospital boards are frequently self-perpetuating, they often seek new members who have backgrounds and philosophies similar to those of existing members. Thus, a board tends to develop a composite personality, and it is important that the CEO be compatible with that personality.

It is equally important that a CEO be able to deal effectively with staff physicians. At any given time, the CEO may have one or more staff physicians who are disaffected by some condition, practice, or requirement of the hospital that the physicians believe adversely affects patient care. The CEO often becomes the lightning rod for the physicians' ire. The CEO must be able to deal diplomatically with distressed physicians. Maintaining a cordial relationship with all the members of the medical staff will be one of the CEO's constant challenges.

Compensation is a key issue in attracting and retaining a CEO. The hospital must be willing to offer a compensation package that is approximately equal to what the candidate could earn if employed in a business establishment of comparable size. The salary and fringe benefits should be sufficient to reflect the individual's contribution to the success of the institution and for that person to enjoy a standard of living comparable to that enjoyed by his or her peers in business. Tax laws impose certain restraints in the design of compensation packages by exempt hospitals and generally require that the overall compensation be reasonable.

The appointment of a search committee by the board chair is usually the first step. This committee should include both members of the board and representatives of the medical staff to enhance the success of the process. Because of the importance of the appointment, the retention of a health care executive recruitment organization should be seriously considered, especially by smaller institutions that may not have the experience or resources to conduct the search without assistance. Recruitment firms generally charge a flat fee plus expenses for their services and continue to provide candidates for interviews until one is selected. The fee is usually about 30 percent of first-year compensation.

Some care should be given to the selection of an executive recruitment firm. It should be large enough to effectively cover as large a geographical area as may be necessary to find the person you are looking for. As firms get larger, however, they will have conducted searches for many hospitals that could have candidates you would like to interview. Does the firm's relationship with those hospitals prevent them from being able to approach candidates they employ? Before you retain a search firm, you should know what limitations there may be on its ability to interview candidates. And before you pay your money up front—which is customary—you should know precisely what the contractual undertaking of the recruiter is. Does it guarantee it will find you an acceptable candidate? It should.

The costs of the candidate's transportation and other expenses in connection with the interview should be borne by

the hospital. In addition to being interviewed by the committee, the candidate should be given an opportunity to tour the
hospital and to meet privately with selected department heads
as well as with a physician group representative of the medical staff. The search committee should have the benefit of
any impressions these individuals may have formed about the
candidate.

A job description for the position should be reviewed
with the candidate before a firm offer is made. This job
description should include the title of the position (president,
executive director, and so on) and should state whether or not
board membership is included. The nature of the responsibilities of the position and the relationship with members of the
board strongly favor inclusion of the CEO as a member of
the board.

The board should consider offering the successful candidate an employment contract for a specified term. By the
time the search procedure is completed, the hospital will have
a substantial investment in the candidate it chooses. An employment contract would help to stabilize the relationship
and protect that investment. From the new CEO's point of
view, the contract should be structured to provide some mea-
sure of employment security. A good form of contract is an
evergreen contract that extends, for example, for a term of one
or more years and is then automatically renewed from year to
year, unless either party gives notice of intention to terminate
sixty or ninety days before the expiration date. The notice
provision allows the hospital some lead time in beginning
another search. The contract should be terminable at any
time for cause.

Caution: Do not get into an adversarial posture with
your new CEO over contract terms. Make it an informal letter
agreement devoid of legalities.

Retaining the CEO

It is important for the governing board to stand behind the
CEO in the execution of his or her duties. This is a difficult,

stressful role that involves long days and nights. The CEO's performance will be improved by a supportive governing board. If the board reaches the point where it feels it can no longer be supportive of the CEO, it is time to make a change in that position.

The chief executive should be subject to an annual performance and salary review. This is usually conducted by a small committee of the board, which reports the results (often in a generalized way) to the board. A form should be devised to rate the CEO on various areas of accountability. The seven principal areas of responsibility that have been suggested as the main concerns of a hospital chief executive are planning and organizing, achieving hospital objectives, quality of care, allocation of resources, crisis resolution, compliance with regulations, and promotion of the hospital.[1]

Although the generality of the following characteristics somewhat limits their usefulness, they do provide a matrix for developing questions that bear on a wide spectrum of board concerns about its CEO. The questions the board evaluation committee should ask would be institution specific, but they might include, among others, the following:

> *Planning and Organizing.* Have the mission statement and the long-range strategic plan been kept up to date? Have the long-range and short-range plans for the institution been followed? Have major needs of the institution, such as building and remodeling and acquisition or replacement of capital equipment, been anticipated so as to permit inclusion in the capital budget?
>
> *Achieving Hospital Objectives.* Are goals with respect to patient days and length of stay being reached? Are relations with the medical staff harmonious and are the goals for medical staff development being achieved? Is fundraising at projected levels? Are new medical services on schedule? Are construction goals being met and capital equipment needs satisfied? Are department head positions filled and all departments adequately staffed?

Quality of Care. How do mortality and morbidity rates compare with those of other institutions providing similar types of services? Is there a system for quality evaluation in place that gives the chief executive and the board the best data available to evaluate the quality of health care delivered, weighted to reflect age, acuity, and the like? What has the institution's experience been with respect to the number of claims filed and the payment of claims made against it?

Allocation of Resources. How close is the institution to projected budget when weighted to reflect changes from projected patient days? Are cost-containment measures being effectively carried out? How many full-time-equivalent employees per adjusted patient day does the institution have when compared with other similar institutions in its area and throughout the country? Do construction programs involve cost overruns? Is an effort being made to improve the institution's administrative techniques and practices to make them more efficient and cost effective?

Crisis Resolution. Have relations between the CEO, the board, the medical staff, and various department heads been harmonious? Have the media obtained and published adverse information that could have been headed off by the administration? Have there been employee strikes, lawsuits relating to administration, or disciplinary actions against groups of employees or physicians? Have there been internal occurrences that could not be resolved without board intervention?

Compliance with Regulations. How many deficiencies were noted in the most recent survey by the Joint Commission on Accreditation of Healthcare Organizations (JCAHO) or in the surveys of other accrediting organizations? Have there been problems in retaining Medicare/Medicaid certification? Have citations been received from the state department of health or other regulatory agencies?

Promotion of the Hospital. What has the CEO done to enhance the image of the hospital in the eyes of the public? Has the hospital sponsored any activities that would make the public aware of the institution and the array of its services available to the community?

When the committee has agreed on its evaluation, it should meet with the CEO to review the results. The atmosphere should be cordial, collegial, and nonjudgmental. The discussion should be a constructive dialogue among the members of the committee and the CEO. By listening, as well as talking, members of the committee may, as an additional benefit, be able to perceive some of the infelicities of the operation of the board itself.

It is very likely that the one person who will have the greatest effect on your hospital's viability is the CEO. The chief executive is the full-time embodiment of the power and authority of the board within the institution and the community it serves. Finding and retaining the right person is of paramount importance.

CHAPTER 6

The Committee System
of Governance

This chapter focuses on two key aspects of the role of trustees in hospital governance: the committee system and the review process.

The Committee System

Except when the hospital has a very small board that can act as a committee of the whole, the responsibility for accomplishing the work of the board is usually divided among standing committees. These committees are assigned certain discrete areas of the board's responsibility that they address at committee meetings held between regular board meetings. At board meetings, committee reports are received, reviewed and adopted, modified, or rejected. Rejection of committee reports and recommendations is unusual because members of a committee develop an expertise in the areas of their committees' responsibility, and boards are generally inclined to accept their recommendations.

The committee method of hospital governance ensures that policy matters are reviewed at least twice, once by the appropriate committee and once again by the full board. This dual consideration tends to eliminate hasty or ill-considered board action. Partially offsetting the benefits of dual consideration, however, is the additional time necessary to obtain both committee and board approval and the overlapping efforts of members of the board who are also members of the committee.

Hospital bylaws usually specify the standing committees of the board, the frequency of their meetings, their composition, and their areas of responsibility. A committee may have a narrow area of responsibility, such as a School of Nursing committee, or it may have multiple areas of responsibility, such as a finance, personnel, and planning committee. Committee structure may vary to meet the needs of any given institution. Committee structure may also be affected by board size. It is desirable to have all board members serve on at least one committee. Collectively, the board's committees should cover the entire spectrum of board responsibilities.

Areas of Board Responsibility

Areas of board responsibility will vary from hospital to hospital, depending, among other things, on institutional sponsorship, charter provisions and bylaws, the mission the board has adopted as set forth in its mission statement, and the parameters of its long-range strategic plan. The lowest common denominator of board responsibilities should generally include the following: planning, marketing, finance, quality of care, risk management, medical staff relationships, community relationships, governmental relationships, human resources, board nomination (unless delegated to another body in a restructured or ecclesiastical system), board evaluation, selection and retention of the CEO, evaluation of the CEO, audit, and education.

In addition, the board has general responsibility for oversight of management and assuring itself that the institution is being operated in accordance with applicable laws and regulations.

Delineating areas of board responsibility is not an exact science; in many instances, there are no distinct methods of separating the areas just listed. For example, quality of care and medical staff relationships overlap. Insofar as board responsibility for human resources relates to salary and wage structure, there is also an overlap with regard to financial responsibility.

Assigning Areas of Board Responsibility to Standing Committees

In establishing standing committees, bylaw drafters should combine related functions within a single committee to avoid the problem of multiple committees with jurisdiction over a single area of responsibility. For example, if finance and human resources are included in the same committee, that committee could consider a wage increase that, if the responsibilities were in separate committees, might necessitate review by each committee. Not only would this entail a wasteful duplication of effort, but the possibility of the two committees reaching inconsistent conclusions would exist.

To economize on staff and committee members' time, the number of committees should be kept at the lowest level practicable.

Ad Hoc Committees

In addition to standing committees that deal with continuing problems, hospital boards may, from time to time, appoint ad hoc committees to deal with a single or isolated concern that does not come within the area of responsibility of the standing committees. Ad hoc committees are dissolved when their function has been performed.

Nonboard Committee Members

Unless there is a bylaw provision to the contrary, hospital committees are not limited to board members but may include representatives of the medical or nursing staff, administration, or interested third parties. In fact, in its *Accreditation Manual for Hospitals*, JCAHO requires that the hospital bylaws provide for the inclusion of medical staff members on governing body committees that consider issues affecting the discharge of medical staff responsibilities.[1]

The Executive Committee

If the board has an executive committee, the bylaws frequently provide that this committee may exercise the power of the board when the board is not in session. Except to the extent that its powers are limited by the bylaws, the mandate of the committee may be as broad as that of the entire board.

The executive committee usually consists of relatively few people to facilitate meetings on short notice, and its membership is ordinarily limited to the leadership of the board. It is better practice for the executive committee to meet on call rather than to have regularly scheduled meetings. Its activities should be limited to two types of situations. The first type is one requiring prompt action in less time than it would take to call a special meeting of the full board. The second type involves those matters requiring a high degree of confidentiality, such as the reduction in privileges of an impaired physician or the discharge for cause of a high-level employee. The small number of people involved and their close relationship with the institution should make it less likely that the confidentiality of the subject matter would be breached. With few members and with those few limited to the board leadership, experienced and knowledgeable individuals may take timely action, which facilitates the decision-making process.

Many well-run institutions, however, regularly schedule meetings of their executive committees (which may meet more frequently than their boards). Regularly scheduled meetings of an executive committee create a tendency for the committee to arrogate to itself the functions of the whole board, though. This tendency becomes almost irresistible when the executive committee schedules its meetings more often than those of the board—for example, monthly as compared to quarterly. The board, at its regular meeting, acts as little more than a rubber stamp. The fact that the executive committee meets regularly may lead other board members to believe that issues only reach them after the committee has thoroughly ventilated, and, in most cases, decided them. Consequently, the board is effectively divided into two different categories: those that make decisions (first-class trustees) and those that rubber stamp the decisions (second-class trustees). The latter cannot be effective members of the board.

The temptation to use the executive committee as a super board is strongest where there is a large and unwieldy board that is sharply divided on many issues. The solution, however, may be to reduce the size of the board or take some other corrective action rather than to displace the board with the executive committee.

Meetings: How to Organize and Run Them

One of the principal burdens of hospital board membership is attending time-consuming board and committee meetings. To the extent that board meetings can be expedited, this burden is lessened, the board is able to accomplish its tasks, and there is a greater likelihood that the members present will have adequate time to fully explore the issues presented.

There should be a senior representative of management assigned to staff each standing committee.

At board and committee meetings, reports are made for two different purposes. Some are for informational purposes to keep the board or committee apprised of developments. These reports require no action. The other type of report presents an issue that is submitted for acceptance or rejection. These are so-called action items. *Action items* relate to matters that are not in the ordinary course of the institution's business and that generally go beyond the scope of any delegation of authority by the board to management, to the medical staff, or to any committee of the board.

Whether an agenda matter is informational or an action item, board or committee members should be furnished in advance with the relevant background material they will need in order to ask knowledgeable questions about any informational report and, after adequate discussion, to vote on any action items. The material should be sufficient to accomplish its purposes. An effort should be made to resist furnishing voluminous documentation that will tend to dismay the recipient by its size. When large amounts of documentation are necessary, however, such documentation should be accompanied by an *executive summary*.

Meetings should be started promptly, and participants should have an understanding that the meeting will be adjourned by a particular hour. Most board members have busy schedules, and if the meeting does not adjourn on time, numerous defections will occur as soon as the adjournment hour is passed.

The chair should try to keep the agenda moving crisply and should have some understanding of parliamentary procedure. The purpose of parliamentary procedure is to safeguard majority rule and to protect any minority interests. If there is no minority, there is no need for such protection. For example, if minutes of a prior meeting have been distributed and no one requests any changes, after an opportunity is given to do so, it is senseless to go through the process of calling for a vote on the approval of the minutes. It is obviously adequate for the chair to state that, there being no objections, the minutes are approved and ordered to be filed. The same is true of any other action item to which there is no objection, unless it is the type of resolution that must be certified to a third party such as a bank or insurance company.

In any organization, meetings have a tendency to become stylized and formal. The same order of business is usually followed, and meetings tend to become routinized. The committee or board will find that the reports they receive frequently tend to deal with the minutiae of the organization's activities, while the main thrust of what is happening is not covered. Interest in the subject matter of meetings declines and attendance lags. To avoid this, the board or committee chair should review the proposed agenda with the management representative staffing the committee before it is distributed to ensure that the agenda includes all items that should be covered.

Board meetings can be made more interesting for the participants if they include a brief presentation by a physician or technologist about something innovative or unusual from a medical or technological standpoint that is being done at the hospital. If possible, the speaker should stay after the meeting to discuss the presentation with interested listeners in more detail.

A skillful meeting chair, without wasting time, will try to engage as many attendees as possible for the discussions that take place at the meeting.

An effort should be made to structure the agenda so that there is more than enough time for a thorough discussion of all agenda items within the time allotted. The most productive meetings are often those that complete the formal agenda before the scheduled time for adjournment, so that the committee members can participate in an unstructured discussion about what is going on at the institution. These discussions are often suggested by, though not directly covered in, agenda items.

The Review Process

Most hospital boards work well. But none of them work at optimum efficiency all the time.

The Need for Review

An almost endless number of factors can reduce board efficiency. To catalogue them would be impossible, but some samples may suggest some of the more egregious ones.

If the board is too large, not all members may have an opportunity to have a committee assignment. If, under those circumstances, all are given committee assignments, the number of members will tend to preclude the possibility of meaningful discussion of issues addressed by the committee. This, in turn, will tend to result in unquestioning acceptance of administration proposals and a dilution of the governing board role. When the issue reaches the board level, the same problem will occur. The larger the board, the less the opportunity for discussion and the greater the tendency toward blind acceptance of administration proposals. The process of governance begins to break down.

Another tendency of large boards is to have the governance powers of the board assumed by the executive committee, which, exercising the power of the board when it is not in session, merely reports on its activity to the board at its next meeting. If the executive committee regularly schedules monthly meetings and the board meets only quarterly, the executive committee will almost certainly wield the true power in the hospital. Such a usurpation will result in the board members who are not members of the executive committee being exposed to corporate liability, while removing the power to protect themselves by participation in decisions on which liability may be predicated.

The hospital may have inadequate mechanisms for keeping the board sufficiently informed about hospital activities to enable its members to discharge their responsibilities. Skillfully expurgated board and medical staff committee minutes are unlikely sources of information about situations that require board attention.

The board organization and committee structure may be inappropriate. The responsibilities assigned to various committees and their membership composition and staffing may result in some board areas of responsibility being overemphasized and others slighted or completely ignored.

The board composition may not be appropriate. If there has been no planning on the part of the nominating committee regarding the experiences, skills, and potentialities necessary to improve the board's effectiveness, and if selection has been limited to new members who are merely compatible with those already on the board, an imbalance will occur. If an otherwise appropriate person can provide a relevant skill or ability not already represented on the board, this should, among other factors, strongly suggest consideration for board membership.

The board may have failed to adequately address program trustee development. Board members having slight, if any, knowledge of the institution or how it operates will not be able to favorably influence its actions. Even a trustee who devotes a great deal of time and attention to learning about the operations of the institution will continually confront new facets of its complexity. An ongoing program for trustee education is essential.

Struggles for power among various board members or cliques may emerge. Ideological disagreement may take place. The board may have vested power in older members unwilling to see control pass in an orderly fashion to younger members.

From this, it should be obvious that all boards should undergo a periodic self-review process to enable them to best utilize their talents to serve their institutions and the public.

Self-Review

The concept of hospital boards conducting a self-review of their own organization and activities is relatively new. In an article titled "Appraising Performance at the Top," Richard L. Johnson discusses the need for board evaluation.[2] Johnson notes that board evaluation differs from a CEO's evaluation in that the board must be evaluated, not only on the basis of the performance of individual members, but also on the basis of the effectiveness of the board as a whole. Johnson suggests that two types of inquiries should be made. The first series of inquiries concerns the board's input to policy-making:

- Does the board carry out its responsibilities in the organizational framework outlined in its own bylaws (that is, does the whole board participate in the decision-making process, or does it merely act as a rubber stamp for the executive committee)?
- Have position descriptions been written and followed by the board members, the chairperson, and the chief executive officer?

- To what extent do all trustees exercise their responsibility for providing input into the decision-making process?
- What periodic and formal review is made of the individual trustee performance?
- What periodic and formal review is made of the performance of the chief executive?

The second type of inquiry relates to the appropriateness of policies reached by the board. These output inquiries include the following:

- From a careful review of board minutes, to what extent do the minutes indicate the adoption of timely courses of action?
- To what extent does the regular reporting system provide trustees with a clear picture of the quality of care being given by the hospital?
- Do trustees receive appropriate financial information?
- Can it be demonstrated that the board acts appropriately on the reports it receives?
- Does the board periodically review the objectives and goals of the hospital and determine to what extent performance has met them?

In keeping with increasing expectations for trustee responsibility and accountability, the JCAHO now requires that hospital bylaws include a provision relating to review of the governing body's performance.[3] Also, in 1986, Bader, Umbdenstock, and Hageman, who developed *Keys to Better Hospital Governance Through Better Information*, published a book titled *Board Self-Evaluation Manual*.[4] This manual contains a set of worksheets to enable a hospital board to accomplish each step in the self-evaluation process.

Generally, the authors recommend the adoption of a six-step process:

1. *Gaining Commitment to the Process.* The board's leadership and individual trustees commit to a serious effort of examining and improving performance.
2. *Planning the Process.* Responsibility is generally assigned

to a committee for planning the self-evaluation process, with adequate administrative support from the CEO.

3. *Setting Board Performance Objectives.* Evaluation, by definition, is the measurement of performance against a standard; it is recommended that board self-evaluation assess performance against the goals and objectives each board establishes for itself, as distinguished from the hospital's objectives.

4. *Gathering the Necessary Information.* How effectively do trustees think the board functions in relation to its goals and objectives? Are the board's structure and working process functioning well? Written questionnaires and/or an interview process are used to compile the board's perceptions of its performance.

5. *Discussing and Interpreting the Information.* A retreat exclusively devoted to self-evaluation is the heart of the process. The board discusses the results of the questionnaires or interviews and considers changes that might be necessary to improve performance.

6. *Linking Evaluation and Performance.* Formulate a board work plan. The annual work plan includes the board's new goals and objectives and recommends changes in board operations. The work plan allows the board to become more educated in advance of foreseeable policymaking and decision making. It also allows the board to track implementation of recommended changes in board structure, processes, and relationships.

Bader, Umbdenstock, and Hageman advise that trustee finger pointing can be avoided by having each board member do his or her own self-analysis. Interestingly, they also recommend that the CEO separately evaluate the board and report conclusions.

The worksheets included in the manual provide a step-by-step guide to conducting the evaluation for boards and CEOs.

Trustees should make sure that their institution's bylaws are in compliance with the self-evaluation requirements of the *Accreditation Manual* and that these bylaw provisions are followed.

CHAPTER 7

Board Accountability
and Limitations

The actions of hospital trustees are subject to judicial review and must meet such standards as may be applied by the court. The discretion of trustees is subject to legislative, judicial, and regulatory constraints.

Trustee Accountability:
The Sibley Memorial Hospital Case

The opinion of Judge Gerhard Gesell of the U.S. District Court for the District of Columbia in the *Sibley Memorial Hospital* Case[1] provides some guidelines as to common law standards for trustee conduct and legal accountability. Because this is the only appellate case we have found that sets forth common law standards for hospital governing board members, its importance merits a rather detailed review.

This suit was brought as a class action by former patients against the defendant corporation as owner and operator of the Sibley Memorial Hospital in Washington, D.C., and against five of its directors and certain financial institutions on whose boards the defendant directors served.

From the early 1950s until 1968, the affairs of the hospital were handled almost exclusively by Dr. Orem, the administrator, and Mr. Ernst, the treasurer. In 1960, when a new hospital building was opened, the bylaws were revised to provide for a board of twenty-five to thirty-five trustees who were to meet at least twice a year. Between such meetings, an executive committee was to represent the board and was authorized to open checking and savings accounts, approve the hospital budget, renew mortgages, and enter into contracts.

A finance committee was created to review the budget and to report regularly on the amount of cash available for investment. Management of those investments was to be supervised by an investment committee.

Despite the 1960 bylaw revisions, the administrator and the treasurer continued to dominate the board. The treasurer made all investment decisions. The executive committee routinely ratified the administrator's and treasurer's actions, and the finance and investment committees had no meetings until 1971, three years after the administrator's death.

After the administrator's death, the chairman of the board and president of the hospital became more active in its day-to-day affairs. The chairman, who was one of the defendants, decided to reactivate the finance and investment committees, but the treasurer continued to exercise control over investment decisions and on several occasions refused to respond to inquiries by other trustees into such matters. It was not until the treasurer's death in 1972 that the other trustees assumed an identifiable supervisory role in the investment policy and fiscal management of the hospital.

The thrust of the former patients' complaint was that a large part of Sibley's investable funds were, and for many years had been, in non-interest-bearing demand-deposit accounts at local banks and financial institutions. Numerous improprieties were claimed in relationships between trustees, financial institutions, and financial advisers. The plaintiffs presented two theories in support of trustee liability. The first theory claimed that the defendants and the financial institutions were part of a conspiracy to enrich themselves at the expense of the hospital. This initial theory was dismissed.

The plaintiffs' second theory in support of trustee liability was that the defendant trustees had breached their duty to Sibley by mismanagement, nonmanagement, and self-dealing.

Before passing on these contentions, Judge Gesell noted that hospital trustees are held to the legal standards for corporate directors rather than the higher standards imposed on trustees of trust estates: "Directors of charitable corporations are required to exercise ordinary and reasonable care in the performance of their duties, exhibiting honesty and good faith. . . . Directors of charitable corporations may delegate investment decisions to a committee of the board so long as all directors assume the responsibility for supervising such committees' work. . . . A director whose failure to supervise permits negligent mismanagement by others to go unchecked has committed an independent wrong against the corporation."[2]

Judge Gesell went on to note that, while there is no bar to placing hospital funds in a bank that has an interlocking directorate with the institution, such transactions are subject to close scrutiny to ensure that the trustees' duty of loyalty has not been violated. Directors should not only disclose any interlocking responsibilities but should also refrain from voting or otherwise influencing a corporate decision to transact business with a company in which they have a significant interest or control.

Applying these standards, the court found that all five of the defendant directors had breached their fiduciary duties to Sibley. Judge Gesell pointed to the fact that they had been members of the finance and investment committees that had not met in over ten years. All of the defendant trustees at one time or another had approved self-dealing transactions with a financial institution in which they were a director, officer, or shareholder.

Judge Gesell noted, however, that the self-dealing had caused no discernible harm to the institution. The terms of the mortgage loan agreement and the investment advisory agreement were fair to Sibley.

In view of the fact that none of the defendant trustees had benefited personally from their breaches of duty and that during the relevant period the overall operation of the hospital in terms of low costs, efficient services, and quality of patient care had been superior, the judge refused to award damages against the defendant trustees or to order their removal from office. As an alternative, the judge entered an injunction requiring that action be taken by the board to ensure that the types of breach of duty that had occurred in the past would not be repeated. The court's decree required that Sibley's investment policy be reduced to writing and be approved by the board, that each new board member be required to read the court's opinion, that the board receive a financial report prior to each board meeting, and that the audit reports for the corporation be made available to the public for the next five years.

The Twin Duties of Care and Loyalty

The *Sibley* case makes clear that the hospital governing board members owe a duty of care to their hospital, as well as a duty of loyalty. Many states have statutes on the duty of loyalty owed to a nonprofit corporation by members of its governing board. As in the *Sibley* case, this duty is normally satisfied if the affected directors make known the nature of their interest in another entity with which the charitable corporation proposes to deal and do not vote on the matter under consideration or otherwise seek to influence the outcome.

Many state statutes require annual written reports by trustees that disclose any interests in third parties with which the hospital has business relationships. Trustees should ensure that their institutions are complying with state law on these matters as well as with the twin duties imposed by the *Sibley* case.

Critics of this decision have pointed out that it provides only modest deterrents for negligent hospital trustees and relates only to their financial responsibilities.

The Revised Model Nonprofit Corporation Act

In 1987, the American Bar Association adopted the Revised Model Nonprofit Corporation Act. The Model Act adopts the prudent man standard used by Judge Gesell in the *Sibley* case for the conduct of directors of nonprofit corporations. The provisions of the Model Act, with respect to the governing board members' duties of care and loyalty, are consistent with Judge Gesell's opinion.

Board Discretion Is Not Unfettered

The discretion of the hospital governing board in carrying out its responsibilities to the institution and the public is not unfettered. In fact, hospital regulation, particularly by the federal government, has exceeded even that found in socialized systems such as the one in Britain.[3]

Statutes and Regulations

The state constitution and the state corporation law under which the institution was incorporated will impose certain limitations on a hospital's authority. The corporate charter may impose further limitations and will usually set forth the purposes for which the corporation was organized. These purposes will serve as parameters for corporate and board activity. The board's actions must also conform to the provisions of its bylaws.

Additionally, an array of statutes and regulations have sharply narrowed the administrative discretion of the institutions to which they relate. Hospitals are also affected by many general laws concerning such matters as wages, hours, and terms and conditions of employment.

Medicare Conditions of Participation

Conditions of Participation for Hospitals under Medicare as described in the Code of Federal Regulations must be met before a hospital can be eligible as a provider under either Medicare or Medicaid.[4] Except for specialized obstetrical and children's hospitals, few hospitals could survive today without being Medicare providers.

These conditions, which largely duplicate the JCAHO's requirements for accreditation and the licensing provisions of some state health departments, require that a hospital have an effective governing body or the equivalent. The board must establish credentialing criteria for physicians and appoint members of the medical staff in accordance with those criteria. The medical staff must be organized under staff bylaws approved by the board. Conditions exist relating to hospital planning, budgeting, certain responsibilities of the medical staff, nursing services, medical records, the operations of the pharmacy and the dietetic department, and the provision of radiological and laboratory services.

Medicare Conditions of Participation for Hospitals have come to represent the lowest common denominator of acceptable hospital organization and operation.

Certificate of Need—Rate Review

Pursuant to the National Health Planning and Resources Development Act of 1974, as amended,[5] nearly all states enacted legislation requiring the issuance of *certificates of need (CON)* for substantial new construction or new medical programs, and a substantial number of states have rate-setting or rate-review requirements for hospitals. The federal mandate for CONs and the availability of federal funds for planning ended in 1986, but many states have retained their CON laws.

The State Health Department

Most state health departments enforce state statutes relating to hospital organization and operations and have adopted regulations relating to hospital operations and health care delivery in their jurisdictions.

States are also responsible for administering federal aid programs, licensing facilities and the professionals who practice in them, and making and enforcing regulations with respect to health and safety.

Accreditation

The JCAHO imposes standards on hospital organization and activities. Failure to substantially comply with these standards will prevent a hospital from obtaining or retaining accreditation.[6] Failure to retain accreditation could adversely affect the hospital's continuing status as a provider under Medicare and Medicaid.[7]

Additionally, JCAHO accreditation is necessary to obtain capital financing, to retain graduate medical education programs, and for participation in most managed care programs.

If the hospital has any long-term debt, the loss of accreditation would almost certainly breach one of the covenants in its mortgage indenture, which requires that the borrowing hospital maintain its accreditation while the loan is outstanding.

Medicare Fraud and Abuse

To protect the financial integrity of the Medicare and Medicaid systems, a variety of federal and state laws provide criminal and civil sanctions for hospitals, physicians, and others who engage in fraudulent or abusive practices affecting the programs. Increased awareness of the cost of such practices to the programs in particular and the industry generally has prompted legislators and enforcement agencies in more recent years to strengthen and enforce these laws. One estimate of the annual total cost of fraudulent activities to the health care industry is $15 billion to $37.5 billion. Commonly termed "fraud and abuse" or "antikickback" laws, they outlaw such practices as payments for patient referrals, billing for unperformed procedures, and physician investments in clinical laboratories. Their broad interpretation by the courts, however, has also raised concerns in the health care industry that many beneficial and common arrangements are technically illegal. For example, partnership distributions by a hospital staff physician joint venture to own and operate a MRI unit could be construed as an illegal payment for the referral of patients by the physician-investors. The potential risk of criminal prosecution or exclusion from the Medicare and Medicaid programs may also have a chilling effect on the proliferation of physician-owned facilities and services that compete with those of the hospital.

Because the laws in this area continue to evolve, hospital trustees must be mindful of their impact on the assessment of various proposals for implementing new services such as joint ventures and physician-recruiting arrangements. These are areas in which the assistance of legal counsel is essential.

The Indenture

If the hospital has long-term debt, it will likely have executed a mortgage indenture that may severely limit the discretion of the governing board to transfer the hospital's assets, undertake additional borrowings, or amend any of its organic documents, such as its charter or bylaws, without obtaining the consent of the lender.

Antitrust

Since 1976, antitrust problems in the health care field have become important enough that all trustees should have some idea of what the antitrust laws provide and how they affect their hospital's activities.

Antitrust law is a complex legal field practiced by lawyers with special knowledge and experience. The purpose of this discussion of the antitrust laws as they affect hospitals is not to make an antitrust lawyer out of the reader, but to make the reader generally aware of antitrust issues and of when to call on antitrust counsel for advice.

The purpose of the antitrust laws is to try to eliminate artificial restraints on the operation of competitive forces in the marketplace. These laws are intended to ensure that those engaged in trade are given full opportunity to compete with each other on the basis of price, quality, service, and reputation.

Some types of antitrust activities, such as price fixing and dividing markets into exclusive territories, are deemed by the courts to be so patently in violation of the antitrust laws as to preclude any need for a factual examination to determine their anticompetitive effects. These are called *per se* violations. Other less pernicious alleged violations are reviewed on their merits under the so-called rule of reason. Under the *rule of reason,* the court will examine the relative competitive benefits and threats of a particular arrangement.

The antitrust laws of the United States are principally contained in three federal statutes:

The Sherman Act

Section 1 prohibits contracts, combinations, and conspiracies in restraint of trade.[8]

Section 2 prohibits monopolization, attempts to monopolize, and conspiracies to monopolize.[9]

The Clayton Act

Section 13(a) through (f) makes it unlawful to discriminate in price, services, or facilities between different purchasers of commodities of like grade and quality where the effect of such discrimination might be to substantially lessen competition.[10]

Section 3 prohibits exclusive dealing arrangements, tying sales and requirement contracts in the sale of commodities,[11] where the effect may be to substantially lessen competition.[12]

The Federal Trade Commission Act

Section 5 prohibits unfair methods of competition and unfair, deceptive acts or practices.[13]

Federal enforcement of the antitrust laws is carried out by the Department of Justice and by the Federal Trade Commission.

The Department of Justice may enforce the Sherman and Clayton Acts through civil or criminal proceedings. Criminal violations of the antitrust laws are felonies. Individuals (including state attorneys general) may sue for damages under the antitrust laws and have the damages they recover trebled under a provision of the Clayton Act. They may also be awarded counsel fees.

Enforcement of the antitrust laws by the Federal Trade Commission is generally by a civil proceeding before an administrative law judge. If the commission prevails, it may then enter a cease-and-desist order. The commission may also promulgate rules defining unfair or deceptive practices or methods of competition under the Federal Trade Commission Act.

Restraints on trade that implicate the federal antitrust laws must be on goods or services in the flow of interstate or foreign commerce or be local restraints on goods or services that affect interstate or foreign commerce.

Prior to 1975, it was thought that the practice of medicine was exempt from the antitrust laws on the basis that a learned profession such as medicine did not constitute trade or commerce. This view was dispelled by the U.S. Supreme Court in *Goldfarb v. Virginia State Bar*.[14]

Prior to 1976, courts had a tendency to view hospital activities as being local and, for that reason, as not affecting commerce. In that year, however, the Supreme Court in *Hospital Building Co. v. Trustees of Rex Hospital* held that, under certain circumstances, a local hospital restraint could have an effect on interstate commerce.[15]

Following the decision in *Hospital Building Co.*, there have been numerous court decisions applying the antitrust laws to hospitals and other health care providers, with varying results. The following is a list of transactions and occurrences that seem to have most frequently attracted the antitrust lightning bolt:

- A hospital failing to grant, withdrawing, or reducing a physician's medical staff privileges

- A hospital refusing to grant privileges to certain adjunct health care professionals such as podiatrists or chiropractors
- A hospital employing a physician or physician group to provide a service such as radiology, pathology, or anesthesiology on an exclusive basis
- A hospital objecting to the grant of a certificate of need to a competitive institution
- A hospital participating in a provider network or acting in concert with one or more competing institutions to combine services previously provided by those institutions separately
- A hospital participating in an alternative delivery system that (1) may exclude other competitive hospitals, (2) may set fees for its members, or (3) conducts a group buying program for its members
- Hospital mergers

This list is not exclusive, and many of the types of arrangements listed, if examined under the rule of reason, might disclose pro-competitive factors supporting them.

Once again, the reader is not supposed to be an antitrust lawyer, but a person who knows when to request an antitrust lawyer's advice.

CHAPTER 8

Responsibilities in Planning and Marketing

Arguably, the most important role of the hospital governing board is that of planning. This is the core task of relating community need to the institution's ability to deliver health services. Failure to make this interpretation accurately and within the capabilities of the institution will result in a failure of the public trust the board has assumed. The application of conventional hospital planning procedures and sound marketing principles should serve to minimize this risk.

Hospitals have engaged in planning for many years. Originally this planning consisted of *facilities project planning* in response to the requirements of the Hill Burton hospital construction program of the late 1940s and 1950s.[1] "Facilities project planning evolved into *facilities master planning* and then into *institutional* or *strategic planning,* which concentrated on the role the hospital would play in the community and how to implement that role.[2]

Marketing is a newer concept for hospitals and one that was somewhat reluctantly adopted because marketing's commercial overtones seemed to conflict with traditional values of charitable activity. Despite this reluctance, the keen interinstitutional competition that has developed between hospitals in the past decade has caused them numerous marketing concerns. These include how they are positioned in the

83

market for the delivery of their services; how these services are priced in relation to their competitors; and how these services are presented to the public, whether through house organs, paid advertising, or other means.

The Planning Process

The planning process has three important steps. The first step is analysis. This step requires the identification of trends and issues and the evaluation of the impact of these trends and issues on the institution. The second step is the development of the plan. This step articulates the hospital's mission, objectives, and strategic initiatives. The final step is implementation. The implementation step identifies specific objectives, resources, tasks, and a timetable. While the board is responsible for all three steps, it usually delegates the first and last to management.

The board's role is to see that the plan is developed, usually through a committee composed of board, management, and medical staff, and then to adopt the plan. The board controls the plan's implementation by using the budgeting process. Effective information collection and analysis are essential to successful planning.

The Mission Statement

The starting point in the planning process is to either develop or update the hospital's mission statement. To develop the initial mission statement, representatives of the board, the medical staff, and the administration meet over a period of time. They work together to develop a statement that sets forth, in general terms, what the hospital is and where it plans to go.

Norman McMillan, in his *Planning for Survival: A Handbook for Hospital Trustees,* suggests that a mission statement should cover the following points:

- What does the hospital stand for?
- Where is it going?

- What can the hospital afford to do?
- What do patients expect of the hospital?
- What medical procedures is the hospital qualified to perform?
- Whom does the hospital serve?[3]

With hospital restructuring and the development of hospital-sponsored commercial ventures, some CEOs and hospital boards have lost the core vision of why the hospital exists. The development or revision of a mission statement can serve to restore first principles.[4]

The board has the ultimate responsibility for the mission statement. It will, however, be a compromise between the views of the board and those of the medical staff and administration.

The Long-Range Strategic Plan

In conjunction with the preparation of the mission statement, the hospital should conduct a self-audit. The self-audit should give consideration to factors affecting the delivery of services by the hospital. These factors include primary care services; the hospital's utilization patterns by clinical services; the utilization patterns of the hospital's competitors by clinical services; the closing of competitive clinical services at other institutions or any reductions in those services and the addition of new competitive services; and trends in geographical origins of patients and projections of population trends for the hospital's service area, including changes in age cohorts.

The self-audit should analyze the health care programs offered by the hospital. It should start with an analysis of admissions by service area, comparing primary care admissions, specialty medicine admissions, and surgery admissions by subspecialty. The audit should continue with an analysis of the hospital's various health care delivery services, which, for a large general hospital, might include the following:

Cardiac and cardiovascular services
General surgery
Outpatient therapeutic and surgical services
Diagnostic services
Emergency services
Maternal and women's care services
Services to infants and children
Oncology services
Neuroscience services
Geriatric services
Orthopedic/musculoskeletal services
Endocrinology
Gastroenterology
Pulmonary service
Nephrology
Rheumatology
Urology
Dermatology
Trauma

The information gathered in the self-audit should assist the committee in developing a suitable mission statement for the hospital and should help the planning and marketing department to prepare a *long-range strategic plan* for the hospital. This should include specific strategic initiatives that will enable the hospital to attain programmatic and financial goals in the face of decreased sources for reimbursement and mounting competition from other health care providers.

Board Responsibilities in the Planning Process

A hospital trustee is not expected to be a hospital planner. Nonetheless, the governing board has the ultimate responsibility for the adoption and execution of the plans of the institution.

The board's first responsibility is to ensure that the planning process takes place and that the requirements of that process are within the abilities of the members of the administrative staff. If not, the board should consider whether an outside consulting firm should be brought in. Plans should include not only a long-range strategic plan but short-term plans as well, which might simply be in the form of goals adopted at the annual meeting for the ensuing years. These goals should be reviewed annually when new goals are established.

The board's second responsibility is to review and evaluate the product of the planning process. Board members should be able to objectively consider whether the proposed long-range strategic plan represents the best utilization of the institution's assets, whether the long-range plan is appropriate in view of the hospital's resources and the community's needs, and whether the plan's objectives are practicable given the institution's capabilities. The board should also determine whether the long-range strategic plan conforms to and is consistent with the hospital's mission statement. If not, one of them must be amended so the two are consistent.

The third responsibility of the board is to monitor the execution of the long-range strategic plan. This duty should fall primarily to the standing committee that is assigned planning responsibility. The bylaw provision setting forth this committee's duties should, among other things, charge it with overseeing the execution of long-range plans and periodically reporting progress back to the board.

Forces outside the control of management or board may strongly influence the direction of hospital development, however. New appointments to the medical staff may bring within the institution practitioners of extraordinary skill and ability who will develop practices in their disciplines much larger or more sophisticated than those that were envisioned when they were granted staff privileges. Such practices may dramatically enlarge the hospital's service area, particularly if the appeal is to a "fly-in" clientele. The burgeoning of such practices may be sufficient to influence the practice patterns even in large, well-established institutions. Such possibilities should be anticipated by the board. Its monitoring processes should be adequate to signal that such an occurrence is taking place so that the board will have adequate time to react. The reaction will, in all probability, be to make available the additional resources necessary to accommodate the expanded service and aid its growth. If this seems like an opportunistic rejection of planning, we should consider that the planning process is an artificial means of determining what the community's health care needs are. What the community buys by way of health care, as in the case of the expanding service, is a better barometer of these needs than can be artificially developed by the planning process, no matter how well perfected.

Trustees, as part of the planning process, must also monitor the progress of legislative response to the health care crisis and try to anticipate the best strategic response for their institutions to these developments. This is further discussed in Chapter Thirteen.

Obviously, the planning process is a continuous one. The members of the board should insist on receiving periodic progress reports. Further, the members should be given an opportunity to review and discuss these reports.

Healing Versus Teaching: A Planning Responsibility

In addition to the healing function, hospitals also conduct teaching and research activities. In a small hospital, these activities may be conducted by the medical and nursing staffs without any formalized program. In large university-affiliated teaching hospitals, however, there may be many residency programs in various medical specialties and schools for various technical specialties. There may be some tension between the healing and teaching functions and, in all but the most rudimentary programs, competition for resources will exist.

In 1910, the Carnegie Foundation for the Advancement of Teaching published a report titled *Medical Education in the United States and Canada.*[5] Compiled and written by Abraham Flexner and popularly known as the *Flexner Report*, it was a critical survey of medical schools in the United States and Canada. The report concluded that medical schools had been doing a poor job of educating physicians during the previous twenty-five years. A number of the medical schools surveyed were proprietary and dependent on student tuition fees for survival. The Flexner report found that many of these did not even require a high school diploma as an admission requirement and had woefully inadequate laboratories and a dearth of clinical materials for observation and study by the students.

Following the publication of the Flexner report, there was a movement for medical schools to affiliate with hospitals and to be acquired by or to develop affiliations with universities. Many larger hospitals wanting to improve their standards developed medical education programs even without university affiliation. All of this resulted in many hospitals developing education programs in the form of internships. The continual presence of young, well-schooled interns in the hospital improved patient care and raised hospital standards.

Yesterday's intern is today's resident. Historically, interns rotated through the hospital's various clinical services. Today's residents, however, are in training to enter a specific medical specialty such as ophthalmology or internal medicine. The only general medical training residents receive is in one-year or transitional-year residencies that they complete before they enter a specific training course. Otherwise this training takes place in residencies in family medicine, which involve all of the clinical disciplines in which a general practitioner must be trained.

Being a teaching hospital adds prestige to a hospital's reputation. Having a residency program is attractive to staff physicians, who appreciate having a physician available to observe their patients when they are out of the hospital. The utilization of meagerly compensated residents instead of highly compensated attending physicians should result in medical economies. Many physicians derive satisfaction from the experience of serving as teachers. The quality of medical service is thereby enhanced.[6]

The board is responsible for determining the levels at which healing, teaching, and research will take place within the institution. The emphasis to be placed on these elements should be recognized in the planning process.

Marketing

Competition among hospitals to sell their services to the public has led to the adoption of marketing techniques. The use of these marketing techniques to sell services may also have led to the socially more desirable result of increasing the knowledge of available hospital services among disadvantaged segments of the population. Consequently, marketing may have increased hospital accessibility to those in need of hospital services.

Broadly stated, a successful marketing program determines which services provided by an institution are wanted by the public, then communicates the availability of these services in a favorable, practicable manner. This process utilizes the accomplishments of the planning process, including the adoption of the mission statement and strategic plan. The balance of the marketing function sets a competitive price for the hospital's service lines and communicates the availability of these service lines to the public. Although communication may take the form of word of mouth, bulletins, or brochures, these methods of publication usually pale in significance compared to advertising in the print and electronic media.

The governing board should be involved in any decision to begin an advertising program for the institution. The question of spending hospital funds on a paid advertising campaign should be carefully considered. Advertising is expensive and must be purchased on a sustained basis. Although results may improve hospital patient care volume, there may be negative aspects to the campaign. Mass advertising directed at prospective patients may not be effective when it is usually the physician who makes the determination as to what patient services to use and at what hospital. Contributors to the hospital may feel diffident about continuing financial support for what they may perceive to have become a commercial venture. Radio and television stations that have previously supported the hospital with free public service broadcasts may be reluctant to do so when such broadcasts deprive them of revenue derived from airing the same messages as paid advertising. The same dollars spent on a public relations campaign might be more cost effective than advertising and without the downside risks.

If, however, a determination is made to embark on an advertising campaign, the board should not only participate in this decision but should also have an opportunity to review the concept of the campaign and its contents. This review should ensure that advertising is appropriate for the institution and the services being promoted. As is the case with any good advertising campaign, all statements and inferences from those statements must be scrupulously honest so as not to mislead the public.

As part of their efforts to minimize commercial implications and emphasize their community service roles, some hospitals have changed the names of their marketing departments to "Department of Communications and Community Relations."

CHAPTER 9

Ensuring
Fiscal Integrity

Hospital boards are reported to spend more of their time (approximately 30 percent) considering the financial aspects of the institution than on any other area of their responsibility.[1] Since most hospital board members are business or professional people, finance is a field with which they are familiar and feel comfortable. Before board members can grasp the economic realities of hospital operations, however, there are certain concepts they should understand. These include, among others, how the hospital is reimbursed for its services and what other sources of funds are available.

Reimbursement

Early American hospitals were operated for the poor as institutions of purely public charity. Patients were generally unable to pay for their care, and payment was not expected. The expenses of operating these hospitals were met by charitable contributions and often by annual grants from state and local governments. For example, in 1910, state, county, and municipal appropriations provided over 30 percent of the income of private charitable hospitals in Pennsylvania.[2] With the emergence of the modern healing hospital and the admission of members of all levels of society as patients, it became necessary for hospitals to adopt daily rates for treating patients on an inpatient basis. Beginning at about a dollar a day for a ward bed at the turn of the century, these rates increased to about seven dollars a day by the end of World War II. An institutional ambivalence developed, with the hospital playing both a charitable role and operating as a business. While providing free ward care to the indigent, the hospital had escalating rates for paying patients in semiprivate and private rooms.

Although the amounts charged for a ward bed in 1946 seem small today, the cost of a protracted hospital stay was an economic threat to the average family. The mid 1930s saw the development of voluntary health insurance plans to provide indemnification against such contingencies. Under the sponsorship of the American Hospital Association, local Blue Cross plans offered health insurance coverage. Beginning in the 1940s, health insurance, provided by Blue Cross and other insurers, was frequently made available as an employee benefit under collective bargaining agreements between labor unions and employers. Employers that provided health insurance coverage for their union employees by contract often voluntarily extended this same coverage to nonunion employees. In 1938, only 1.5 million Americans had health insurance, but by 1969, over 170 million Americans were covered.[3] In 1965, Medicare and Medicaid were enacted by Congress,[4] greatly increasing the number of people covered by third-party reimbursement, so that today only about thirty million Americans are without such coverage. These thirty million Americans, however, represent the Achilles' heel of the American health care delivery system.

Reimbursement Systems Other than Medicare and Medicaid

Hospitals are paid for their services under a number of different payment or reimbursement systems. The system utilized is determined by the source of payment. Some examples may be helpful.

Patients without any type of insurance coverage, those
who pay their own bills, pay billed charges. *Billed
charges* are what a hospital, other than one in a rate-
review state, decides to bill for its services. Such payers are sometimes said to pay *retail*. This is true also
for those patients who have commercial health insurance coverage with an insurer that has no specific
contractual discount arrangement with the hospital.

Many Blue Cross plans reimburse hospitals for *allowable costs,* costs incurred by the hospital in treating
patients covered by the plan, limited to the costs that
the hospital and the plan have contractually agreed
to include. These are usually substantially less than
billed charges. Any discount from billed charges is
called a *contractual allowance*. This is the term used
to designate the difference between charges and
actual reimbursement, where reimbursement is less
than charges. Such is the case where the hospital has
a Blue Cross contract or a contract with some other
third-party payer that provides for the payment of
something less than charges. Contractual allowances
are also applicable where Medicare or Medicaid payments are less than charges. For instance, it is customary at the top of the income statement to show
gross patient revenue, which represents full charges.
This is reduced by *contractual allowances* and a provision for uncollectible accounts. Uncollectible accounts include both *bad debts* and *charity care*. Gross
patient revenue, as so reduced, is designated *net patient revenue.*

Prepaid health plans such as HMOs and PPOs usually
contract with hospitals for the provision of services to
their members at some discount from billable charges.

Reimbursement Under Medicare and Medicaid

Medicare is administered by the Health Care Financing Administration (HCFA) within the Department of Health and

Human Services. It provides health care for the elderly and the disabled who fall within its coverage.

The Medicare program has two trust funds available for the payment of health care costs, Part A and Part B. Part A is supported by mandatory contributions from employees, employers, and the self-employed and was established to reimburse hospitals, nursing homes, and home health care providers for their reasonable costs in providing inpatient services. Part B was established to reimburse physicians for their usual, reasonable, and customary fees for services provided to covered patients, for hospital-based physician services, and for hospital outpatient services to Medicare patients.

Although Medicare reimbursement was originally based on allowable costs, in 1983, the Social Security Act was amended to introduce a new method of hospital reimbursement. Under this system, reimbursement for most services is by DRGs (diagnostic related groups) that attempt to relate the amount of reimbursement to the severity of the patient's disease as diagnosed at discharge, on a standardized basis. Under the DRG system, the amount of reimbursement is determined on a per-discharge basis by the diagnosis the attending physician assigns to each case. Except where a hospital's cost related to a patient's treatment or length of stay is greater than the norm, the amount of reimbursement for each case assigned to the same DRG is the same. A patient whose treatment or length of stay exceeds established norms (these patients are called *outliers*) will have such excess care reimbursed at a lower rate than reimbursement provided under the DRG. Charges and costs are irrelevant under the DRG system, except that medical education and capital costs are reimbursed separately as pass-throughs on a formula basis that generally provides hospitals with less than their actual costs for these items.

Some services are still cost-reimbursed. Medicare reimburses hospitals for 80 percent of the allowable cost for outpatient services and for psychiatric, rehabilitation, and substance abuse treatment. The patient is responsible for the other 20 percent.

The Medicaid program, originally enacted at the time

of the Medicare program, reimburses for hospital and medical care for the eligible needy. The program is financed by state and federal funds; it is administered by the individual states, and each state determines its own reimbursement policy. Reimbursement for services varies with the different states, but it is generally cost-based reimbursement or may be some form of *prospective payment system (PPS)* similar to DRGs. Medicaid reimbursement in most states is less than costs.

Sources of Revenue

The sources of a hospital's operating revenues include per diem charges for routine inpatient services, charges for outpatient services, and charges for ancillary services such as the use of the operating rooms, anesthesia, laboratory fees, and the like. These will not be applicable to DRG cases and will be reduced by *contractual allowances* given to some third-party payers.

The hospital may also receive income on endowment funds held by it or for its benefit and from contributions received from the public. Many hospitals, especially those that have been restructured, have established or acquired businesses, usually operated by affiliated corporations, to develop streams of income other than traditional patient care sources.

Hospitals may receive government grants, usually earmarked for a particular purpose, or contributions from individuals, decedents' estates, trusts, and charitable foundations.

Limitations on Revenue Enhancement

There are limitations on a hospital's ability to enhance its revenues from patient care by increasing room rates and charges for ancillary services. If the hospital is in a rate-review state, it may be unable to obtain approval for a requested increase in its room rates and other charges. Even if it is not in a rate-review state, the effect on hospital revenues of an increase in room rates or other charges is reduced geometrically by the fact that most of the hospital's reimbursement usually comes from third-party payers who do not pay charges. For example, if a hospital's patient mix is 50 percent Medicare (DRGs and allowable costs), 25 percent Blue Cross (allowable costs), and only 25 percent commercial insurance or private pay (charges), a room rate increase would only affect the last category and would have to be four times the amount that would have been necessary if it had applied to all payers.

Cost Shifting

Medicaid reimbursement is usually substantially less than the hospital's costs in providing services to Medicaid patients. Because Congress continues to decrease reimbursement for such patients, hospitals are increasingly suffering losses in caring for these categories of patients. Planned care providers like HMOs and PPOs usually contract with hospitals to provide services at a discount. This means that the hospital will have to shift the unreimbursed costs of caring for its Medicare and Medicaid patients and possibly HMO and PPO patients to some other category, usually the private payers and commercial insurance carriers who pay charges. This is discussed in Chapter One.

Accounting Methods

Hospital financial reports are similar to those prepared for business corporations, with some notable exceptions. For instance, if the hospital has endowment funds that have been restricted by the donor to a specific purpose, the hospital will follow fund accounting principles in the preparation of its balance sheet. In fund accounting, all unrestricted funds are reported as the *general fund*. All donor-restricted funds are accounted for separately in three categories: funds for a specific purpose, either operating or capital, and endowment funds.

Occasionally, a hospital board, to ensure that funds will

be available to accomplish a specific objective, will designate certain funds to be used for that purpose. These are referred to as *board-designated funds*. Although board-designated funds are not available to management for use except for the designated purpose, the board may, at its discretion, remove or change such designation. Therefore, board-designated funds are accounted for as part of the general fund.

A hospital's financial statements include the following: general funds comparative balance sheet, comparative statement of revenue and expense, restricted funds comparative balance sheet, and statement of cash flows. The *general funds comparative balance sheet* (Table 1) sets forth the assets, liabilities, and fund balances for the general fund. The *restricted funds balance sheet* (Table 2) does the same for the restricted fund. The *comparative statement of revenue and expense* (Table 3) separately states operating and nonoperating revenue. Patient service revenue is shown first, reduced by contractual allowances and uncollectible accounts to arrive at net patient service revenue. The addition of other operating revenue results in a figure for total operating revenue. From this is deducted total operating expenses to come up with income from operations. Nonoperating revenue is then added to this to arrive at excess of revenue over expense. The *Statement of Cash Flows* (Table 4) provides the reader with a conversion of accrual accounting to a cash basis and ultimately indicates the change in cash position of the organization from the beginning to the end of the accounting cycle. This statement also breaks down the cash position changes as (1) related to operations, (2) related to investments, and (3) related to financing activities.

In the comparative statement of revenue and expense, bad debts and uncompensated care are reported as reductions in patient service revenues. Under generally accepted accounting principles, they would be reported as an expense.[5]

With the exceptions noted above, hospitals follow generally accepted accounting principles. In applying these principles, hospitals utilize the *Hospital Audit Guide*.[6]

Table 1. Pillhaven Hospital General Funds Comparative Balance Sheet.

Assets	Dec. 31, 1990	Dec. 31, 1989
Current assets		
Current operating funds:		
Cash and short-term investments	$ 3,500,000	$ 3,000,000
Accounts receivable:		
Patients	62,000,000	59,000,000
Less estimated allowances:		
Doubtful accounts	4,000,000	3,500,000
Contractual adjustments	30,000,000	28,000,000
Total allowances	34,000,000	31,500,000
Net accounts receivable	28,000,000	27,500,000
Other receivables	2,000,000	1,700,000
Inventories	900,000	800,000
Prepaid expenses	1,200,000	1,400,000
Total current assets	35,600,000	34,400,000
Assets whose use is limited:		
Funds held by bond trustees	65,000,000	85,000,000
Funded depreciation	22,000,000	18,000,000
Malpractice self-insurance trust	4,000,000	3,500,000
Total assets whose use is limited	91,000,000	106,500,000
Other assets	1,700,000	1,600,000
Bond conversion costs	1,900,000	1,900,000

Liabilities and Fund Balance	Dec. 31, 1990	Dec. 31, 1989
Current liabilities:		
Accounts payable	$ 4,500,000	$ 5,000,000
Accrued employment costs	6,000,000	5,500,000
Other accrued expenses	7,500,000	7,000,000
Due to third parties	6,000,000	6,500,000
Current portion of long-term debt	4,000,000	4,400,000
Total current liabilities	28,000,000	28,400,000
Deferred revenue	1,700,000	1,600,000
Self-insurance liability	1,500,000	1,400,000

Property, plant, and equipment:		
Land and land improvements	5,500,000	5,500,000
Buildings, improvements, and fixed equipment	71,000,000	69,000,000
Movable equipment	51,000,000	46,000,000
Construction in progress	28,000,000	8,000,000
Total fixed assets	155,500,000	128,500,000
Less: accumulated depreciation	55,500,000	49,500,000
Net property, plant, and equipment	100,000,000	79,000,000
Total assets	$230,200,000	$223,400,000

Long-term debt	110,000,000	113,000,000
Total liabilities	141,200,000	144,400,000
Fund balances	89,000,000	79,000,000
Total liabilities and fund balance	$230,200,000	$223,400,000

Table 2. Pillhaven Hospital Restricted Funds Comparative Balance Sheet.

	Dec. 31, 1990	Dec. 31, 1989
Assets		
Specific-purpose funds		
Cash	$ 800,000	$ 700,000
Investments	4,200,000	3,900,000
Other receivables	1,000,000	800,000
	6,000,000	5,400,000
Endowment fund		
Investments	3,000,000	2,800,000
Total assets	$9,000,000	$8,200,000
Liabilities and fund balances		
Specific-purpose funds		
Other accrued expenses	400,000	300,000
Fund balance	5,600,000	5,100,000
	6,000,000	5,400,000
Endowment fund		
Fund balance	3,000,000	2,800,000
Total liabilities and fund balances	$9,000,000	$8,200,000

Table 3. Pillhaven Hospital General Funds Comparative Statement of Revenue and Expense.

	For the years ended	
	Dec. 31, 1990	Dec. 31, 1989
Revenue from patients:		
Inpatient routine	$ 88,000,000	$ 65,000,000
Inpatient ancillary	172,000,000	130,000,000
Outpatient	40,000,000	28,000,000
Gross patient revenue	300,000,000	223,000,000
Deductions from revenue:		
Contractual allowances	(165,000,000)	(110,000,000)
Other allowances	(10,000,000)	(7,000,000)
Total deductions	(175,000,000)	(117,000,000)
Net patient revenue	125,000,000	106,000,000
Other operating revenue	3,000,000	2,500,000
Total operating revenue	128,000,000	108,500,000

Table 3. Cont'd.

	For the years ended	
	Dec. 31, 1990	Dec. 31, 1989
Operating expenses:		
Salaries and wages	52,000,000	44,000,000
Physician salaries and fees	5,500,000	5,000,000
Employee benefits	10,800,000	8,000,000
Purchased services	3,200,000	3,400,000
Medical/surgical supplies	20,000,000	16,000,000
Drugs and intravenous solutions	5,000,000	4,000,000
Utilities and maintenance	4,400,000	3,600,000
Other supplies and expenses	9,400,000	8,200,000
Insurance	2,200,000	2,000,000
Depreciation	6,000,000	7,000,000
Interest	1,500,000	1,800,000
Total operating expenses	120,000,000	103,000,000
Income from operations	8,000,000	5,500,000
Nonoperating revenue	2,000,000	1,500,000
Excess of revenue over expense	$10,000,000	$7,000,000
Patient days	135,000	131,000
Admissions	17,000	16,500

Table 4. Pillhaven Hospital Statement of Cash Flows.

	Twelve Months Ended Dec. 31, 1990
Operating activities and nonoperating revenue	
Excess of revenue over expense	$10,000,000
Adjustments to reconcile excess of revenue over	
expense to net cash provided by operating	
activities and nonoperating revenue:	
Depreciation	6,000,000
(Increase) decrease in patient accounts	(500,000)
receivable	
(Increase) decrease in other receivables	(300,000)
(Increase) decrease in other current assets	100,000
(Increase) decrease in other assets	(100,000)
Increase (decrease) in accounts payable,	500,000
accrued employment costs, and other	
accrued expenses	
Increase (decrease) in net amounts due to	(500,000)
third-party payers	

Table 4. Cont'd.

Twelve Months Ended Dec. 31, 1990	
Increase (decrease) in current portion of long-term debt	(400,000)
Increase (decrease) in deferred revenue	100,000
Increase (decrease) in self-insurance liability	100,000
Net cash provided by operating activities and nonoperating revenue	15,000,000
Investing activities	
Assets whose use is limited:	
Funds held by trustee under bond indentures	20,000,000
Funded depreciation	(4,000,000)
Malpractice self-insurance trust	(500,000)
Purchase of property and equipment	(27,000,000)
Net cash used by investing activities	(11,500,000)
Financing activities	
Repayment of long-term debt	(3,000,000)
Net cash used by financing activities	(3,000,000)
Increase in cash and cash equivalents	500,000
Cash and cash equivalents at beginning of period	3,000,000
Cash and cash equivalents at end of period	$ 3,500,000

The New Health Care Audit Guide

The American Institute of Certified Public Accountants (AICPA) has been working on revisions to the *Hospital Audit Guide* since 1982. Guided by its Health Care Committee, the AICPA undertook a lengthy and thorough process for developing the revised guide, seeking public input and approvals from the Auditing Standards Board (ASB), the Accounting Standards Executive Committee (AcSEC), the Financial Accounting Standards Board (FASB), and the Governmental Accounting Standards Board (GASB). These efforts culminated in July 1990 with the issuance of *Audits of Providers of Health Care Services* (hereafter referred to as *the guide* or the *new guide*). The new guide is effective for fiscal years beginning on or after July 15, 1990.

Some of the major changes resulting from the new guide are summarized as follows.

Patient Service Revenues. Hospitals have historically reported revenues from patient services at the gross charge level on the statement of revenues and expenses and then deducted contractual discounts, bad debts, and charity care dollars to arrive at net patient revenues. The new guide calls for a reporting of only the net patient revenues on the face of the financial statements, with disclosure of revenue deductions as an option in the notes to the financial statements.

Charity Care. The new guide requires that service charges related to charity care be excluded from gross revenue. Charity care implies that no payment is expected for services rendered, and according to FASB's Concepts Statement No. 6, when services are rendered without the expectation of cash inflow, revenues should not be considered as earned.

Bad Debts. Bad debts are considered to be losses resulting from the extension of credit to a patient who is able but unwilling to pay. The new guide requires that bad debts be reclassified as an operating expense rather than a revenue deduction, as was previously the treatment.

Nonoperating Revenues. Prior to issuance of the new guide, certain revenues not associated with patient services—such as investment income, contributions, and so on—were categorized as nonoperating revenue and shown on the financial statement below the income from operations line. Under the rules, these revenues, with a few exceptions, will be reclassified as other operating revenue, to be consistent with FASB Concepts Statements No. 5 and No. 6.

The new audit guide contains other, more subtle, changes and should be read by those who have a detailed interest in hospital financial statement format and disclosure.

Accounting Inadequacies

In one very material respect, hospital accounting has proven to be inadequate. Large corporate purchasers of health care believe that hospitals should be able to develop cost accounting systems that will enable purchasers to identify revenues and costs for each service the hospital provides. This information, when matched with the medical outcome of treatment of a statistically valid sample of cases in a particular service, would give such a purchaser an idea of the comparative cost-effectiveness of services provided by an institution on a service-line by service-line basis. When combined with data on acuity of illness, morbidity, mortality, and so on, this information would enable a purchaser of services to determine whether a particular institution is delivering cost-effective quality health care, especially in comparison with other institutions collecting data on the same basis.[7] In Pennsylvania, where there is a Health Care Cost Containment Council, the council has mandated use of the MedisGroups system by hospitals for preparing the statistical data the council requires hospitals in Pennsylvania to file on a regular basis. How the quality of care in a hospital setting can be accurately quantified is not fully understood, and efforts are being made to develop new computer programs to make quality of care susceptible to more precise definition and measurement.

Operating and Capital Budgets

Each year the hospital prepares operating and capital budgets that require the board's approval. This is a process that involves months of staff time. Before the proposed budgets are presented to the relevant board committees and ultimately to the board itself, the chief executive officer, the chief operating officer, and the chief financial officer spend a great deal of stressful time in each other's company.

Operating and capital budgets serve somewhat different purposes. The *capital budget* is largely a planning tool and a device that enables the hospital to identify sources of funds to meet large capital expenditures. The *operating budget,* on the other hand, is used mainly for operating control purposes.

The first responsibility of the board with respect to the budgets is to determine whether they are consonant with the mission statement and long-range strategic plan of the hospital. Assuming that they are consonant, the next step is to determine the validity and reasonableness of the underlying assumptions on which the budgets are based. Is the operating budget consistent with the budgets for prior years? If there is a departure from the figures for prior years, does this reflect the results of a trend, the provision of a new health service, or the discontinuance of an existing one?

The board's review of proposed budgets should be searching and vigorous. Initially, this review should involve the board committee that is responsible for financial matters. Once it has gotten past this committee, it should be subject to a thorough reexamination at the board level.

During the period an operating budget is in effect, the board should have a chance to analyze how close actual financial performance has been to the budget. This information should be included in periodic financial statements presented to the board and reviewed at its regular meetings. Unforeseen financial events may and probably will occur, but the board is entitled to receive timely explanations for any material variances between budgeted and actual performance.

Project Financing

Periodically, in fulfilling their missions, hospitals will need to obtain additional capital funds. For example, in communities where the population is expanding, hospitals may need to increase bed capacity. In static communities, where the number of existing hospital beds is adequate (or even excessive), hospitals may need to remodel obsolete facilities, construct facilities to provide new services, or replace capital equipment. The solutions to these types of problems can involve the expenditure of large amounts of money. Obtaining these funds is clearly the responsibility of the governing board.

Today, the largest source of hospital capital by far is borrowed money, usually in the form of tax exempt revenue bonds. While tax exempt financing continues to be the preferred source of hospital capital funds, recent changes in the tax laws have eliminated certain advantages to the issuer of these types of bonds, which has made them less attractive as investments for some institutional buyers. Tax exempt financing is a field that is highly sophisticated and subject to rapid change. Any institution that is considering tax exempt revenue bond financing should obtain the services of a financial adviser with recent and substantial experience in this field.[8]

Although relatively few dollars (about 4 percent of hospital construction costs[9]) are raised by fund development compared to borrowing, the governing board will still find this to be the most expedient way to finance a capital project on occasion.

Conducting a capital fundraising drive is a fine science. Although most of the dollars raised will come from very few sources, the campaign should be as broad as possible. Members of the governing board will know who the potential large contributors are, what approach will appeal to them, and how to get the maximum contributions. Some members of the hospital board may be included among these large contributors. Members of the board will have roots going deep in the community and will know what campaign strategy will be the most effective with members of the hospital's constituency.

Many members of the hospital board will have served on the boards of other charitable corporations, such as schools, colleges, or churches. Hence they will be familiar with other capital campaigns in the community and will know why they succeeded or failed.

Fund Development

It is the board's responsibility to determine whether or not a capital fundraising drive should be conducted and the amount of the goal. The board should also determine whether the campaign should be conducted in-house, using hospital personnel, or if the services of one of the many professional fundraising organizations should be employed. Unless the campaign is a small one with few prospects to be called on, it would be very difficult for a hospital without a professionally staffed fund development office to conduct an in-house campaign.

In fundraising, the CEO of the institution usually takes less of a leadership role and looks more to the board for direction. Unless the CEO grew up in the community served by the hospital or has spent many years at the hospital, he or she will not be as familiar with the social and economic infrastructure of the community as most members of the board.

Annual Giving; Planned Giving

In addition to providing leadership for capital fundraising drives, the board should try to develop an annual giving program. This usually takes the form of a year-end appeal to support a specific need of the institution. It is important to the hospital to encourage as many people as possible to get used to giving regularly in whatever amount they think is appropriate. Not only does this provide financial support for the hospital, but it helps contributors identify with the institution. That is, it becomes their hospital.

For the more affluent members of the hospital's constituency, the board should institute a program for planned (sometimes called deferred) giving. The program should encourage people to leave bequests to the hospital in their wills, to make the hospital the beneficiary of life insurance policies, and to establish other instruments to benefit the hospital, such as *charitable lead trusts, charitable remainder trusts*, and the like. A charitable lead trust distributes a portion of the trust's property to a charity for a fixed period of years, which may be measured by someone's life. At the end of the term, the trust is terminated and the property is distributed to noncharitable beneficiaries. A charitable remainder trust operates the opposite way. A percentage of the property in such a trust is initially distributed to noncharitable beneficiaries until the end of the term. The remainder of the property is then distributed to charity.

Support Foundations

Large hospitals and those serving affluent communities might consider establishing a separately incorporated support foundation. Many hospitals have done this in recent years. The establishment of a support foundation with a separate professional staff puts the hospital's development program on a full-time basis, administered by persons for whom fund development is their only hospital responsibility. Frequently, there are wealthy persons who are unwilling to serve on a hospital board because of the commitment involved or the exposure to potential liability hospital board membership entails. The same persons, however, might be willing to serve on a support foundation board and to become substantial contributors.

By accumulating funds outside the hospital corporation, the hospital may be able to avoid including income earned on these funds in its rate base in a rate-regulation state. This may also protect the funds from attachment in a large tort liability recovery against the hospital.

Investment Management

Any hospital that has endowment or other funds must accept the responsibility for their investment. It is a fundamental responsibility of the governing board to ensure that the institution's funds are invested so that the principal is secure and a fair return is recovered. Even if the governing board includes members who are professional investment advisers, it is usually the wiser course of action to retain the services of someone who is not a board member to perform this function. Board members with investment skills and experience should serve on the board committee having investment responsibility; they should look over the shoulders of the retained advisers to make sure they are doing a good job.

Where hospitals have accumulated large amounts of capital in their plant accounts or endowment funds, they may wish to divide the funds among two or more investment advisers and compare the results of their efforts regularly.

The board should prepare a detailed statement of investment strategy establishing goals and limitations, and this should be given to its investment advisers. The policy should be a conservative one, more concerned about the safety of capital than the generation of income.

CHAPTER 10

Improving Quality for Patients and Staff

In any hospital, improving the quality of care and of board-staff relations are major responsibilities of the trustees.

Improving the Quality of Care

This section touches on quality assurance, risk management, and continuous quality improvement.

Quality Assurance

It is clear from the decision in the *Darling* case that a hospital has corporate responsibility for the quality of health care delivered within the institution and that such responsibility ultimately translates into board responsibility for quality assurance. The continuing neglect of that responsibility would be an independent act of negligence against the institution. Thus, "quality assurance, usually a responsibility of health care practitioners, is intended to identify and resolve problems in patient care and to identify and take advantage of opportunities to improve patient care."[1]

Each patient in the hospital is under the care of a licensed physician or allied health care professional. Any intrusion on that relationship by the board or administration, in the absence of the disability or incompetence of the staff member, would be illegal and inexcusable. Except in extreme cases, the hospital's obligation to monitor the care delivered by physicians within the institution is done in the following ways: by the credentialing process; by the reappointment process, which, according to the JCAHO's credentialing requirements, must take place at least every two years;[2] and by any reports periodically made on behalf of the organized medical staff with respect to its medical care evaluation activities.

Such reports are made to the board committee that is responsible for medical activities in the hospital. The medical staff has a committee charged with responsibility for quality of care on which both the administration and the board should be represented.

The JCAHO's Standard QA.1 requires that each accredited hospital have an "ongoing quality assurance program designed to objectively and systematically monitor and evaluate the quality and appropriateness of patient care, pursue opportunities to improve patient care, and resolve identified problems."[3] This standard sets forth the following requirements:

> QA. 1.1 The governing body strives to assure quality patient care by requiring and supporting the establishment and maintenance of an effective hospital-wide quality assurance program.
>
> QA. 1.2 Clinical and administrative staffs monitor and evaluate the quality and appropriateness of patient care and clinical performance, resolve identified problems, and report information to the governing body that the governing board needs to assist it in fulfilling its responsibility for the quality of patient care.
>
> QA. 1.3 There is a written plan for the quality assurance program that describes the program's objectives, organization, scope, and mechanisms for overseeing the effectiveness of monitoring, evaluation, and problem solving activities.[4]

The board's task is to develop information systems that will provide it with adequate data to make informed judgments about the uniform provision of quality health care throughout the institution. For most hospital boards, the basic medium of exchange of information is the joint conference or medical affairs committee. The information given to this committee usually consists of written minutes of various staff committee meetings, such as those of the staff executive committee, the clinical care committee, the credentials and nominating committee, the planning committee, the education and research committee, and so on. The meeting of the joint conference or medical affairs committee is largely taken up with the chairs of the various committees giving oral summaries of the written minutes previously furnished to the members of the committee. Unfortunately, the least likely place to find any indication that anything in the hospital is amiss is in the written report of any committee. Almost invariably the minutes will relate to routine matters. If anything untoward is discussed at the meeting, the secretary will probably be told not to report it. The bottomless pit of medical and hospital tort liability has conditioned physicians and trustees alike against making gratuitous written statements against either their own, their colleagues', or the hospital's interest.

In 1983, the Hospital Trustee Association of Pennsylvania produced a very useful publication, *Keys to Better Hospital Governance Through Better Information*.[5] This publication argues that by utilizing four "keys," the board can obtain the relevant information necessary to fulfill its responsibilities in various areas of hospital governance. These keys are the following:

- Developing a clear understanding of the board's responsibility in the subject matter (as distinguished from the separate responsibilities of the medical staff and administration)
- Understanding the type and quality of information needed to fulfill the perceived responsibility

- Identifying the process for providing that information
- Adopting formats for providing the information[6]

Keys to Better Hospital Governance Through Better Information illustrates the use of the "keys" technique with respect to various trustee responsibilities, including quality of care, by presenting detailed worksheets appropriate for a step-by-step analysis and resolution of the specific problem.

This publication also points out the need for a quality assurance program to develop trust between the staff physicians and the board members, noting that the physicians' clinical training, experience, and concern for preserving the private practice of medicine bring them to the conference table with a somewhat different perspective than the independent trustees with none of those encumbrances:

> The board's quality assurance role often casts it as a reluctant antagonist of community physicians. Without clinical training, good data, or executive leadership, trustees are asked to look over the shoulders of prideful professionals who bear the responsibility of caring for their patients and sustaining a profitable practice. One of two scenarios usually results. In many hospitals delegation becomes abrogation as trustees opt to leave quality issues in the hands of the doctors. At the other extreme, some boards and medical staffs come to loggerheads over issues of quality or medical economics, each claiming to represent the best interests of patients and the community.
>
> Non-productive confrontation can be avoided, or turned into productive conflict and cooperation— but only if trustees, physicians, and management work together to build an environment of trust.[7]

Risk Management

Risk management is a hospital program intended to protect its financial assets from loss by ensuring adequate funding of liability for perceived risks through insurance coverage, by taking steps to reduce liability if an event giving rise to liability should occur, and by trying to reduce the occurrences of those events that are most likely to lead to liability.[8]

Although quality assurance does not entirely include risk management, they overlap enough to warrant management's consideration of the integration of the two programs for administrative purposes.[9]

Generally, risk management deals with departures from acceptable standards of care toward the institution's patients, employees, or members of the public that result in injury and that may entitle the injured party to monetary damages. Even without a departure from standards of care, risk management may be concerned with the need for the institution to defend itself against an entirely unmeritorious claim.

Risk management involves identifying and controlling exposure to loss both before and after the event giving rise to liability occurs.

Health care providers today are at increased risk for malpractice liability for a number of reasons. The standard of medical care is rising as technology improves; also, the locality rule, which held health care providers only to local standards of care, has largely been replaced by higher uniform national standards. Moreover, doctors are no longer reluctant to testify against other doctors or hospitals, and the end of the eleemosynary defense has exposed nonprofit hospitals to tort liability. Finally, legal decisions such as *Darling* have imposed new types of liability on hospitals.

Most large hospitals have a senior staff person whose primary responsibility is risk management. Such a hospital will have written risk management and quality assurance plans.[10] The *risk management plan* will provide for the completion of an incident report for every unusual occurrence in the institution that may result in a claim for damages. James E. Orlikoff reports that a 400-bed metropolitan community hospital will average sixteen malpractice suits a year and that there will be approximately 3,600 incident reports filed during that period, for a ratio of 225 incident reports to each lawsuit.[11] Orlikoff distinguishes between incidents that are custodial related (slip and fall) and those that are medically related, such as a missed diagnosis or an unplanned return to surgery. Custodial-related claims are more numerous statistically than those that are medically related but usually involve much smaller recoveries. Medical occurrences are likely to be costly and are seldom the subject of an incident report, since they are unknown when they occur.

Hospitals may obtain insurance to protect their assets from liability claims and also from the expense of defending against such claims. Insurance costs, however, have skyrocketed in the past twenty years. A hospital that in the mid 1960s paid no more than $10,000 in premiums for all of its insurance coverages might today pay a hundred times that amount, or $1,000,000. In view of the great expense of insurance premiums, a hospital with a good safety record, if it is able to qualify, might elect to become self-insured or, alone or with others, might establish its own captive insurance carrier. Self-insured hospitals will often obtain insurance coverage for limits of liability in excess of the amounts they are willing to assume. First dollar insurance coverage is the most expensive. The premium per dollar of coverage usually decreases as the dollar amount of retained risk increases.

Hospitals wanting to become self-insurers will probably have to obtain the approval of their state department of health, state insurance commissioner, or both. Most states will require hospitals to establish and maintain substantial trust funds for the benefit of their claimants as a condition to permitting them to self-insure.

The board should see to it that the hospital has risk management and quality assurance plans in effect. An identifiable member of the administration should serve as *risk manager* and be responsible for both plans' execution. The board should periodically receive reports relating to claims made against the hospital, claims paid, and steps taken to reduce exposure, and the board should be provided with an opportunity to review these matters with the *claims manager* at regular intervals. The question of insurance or self-insurance should also be reviewed, from time to time, in light of the institution's experience and changes in the insurance market.

Board members, for their own security, should find out whether the hospital has directors' and officers' (D&O) liability insurance coverage. This insurance coverage is expensive, difficult to obtain, and usually excludes certain major risks, such as antitrust and statutory liability. Board members should also make sure that the hospital bylaws contain an indemnification provision that gives members of the governing board (and all employees and agents) the maximum protection permitted under the state's nonprofit corporation act.

There is one factor that is important to both quality assurance and risk management: patient satisfaction. Patients' perceptions that they have received good care are important. Board members should have some means of monitoring levels of patient satisfaction and should try to see that this is maintained at as high a level as possible. Satisfied patients are not likely to make claims, irrespective of treatment outcome.

Continuous Quality Improvement

A potential new imperative for hospitals has recently been evolving. In addition to quality assurance, hospitals are becoming concerned with *continuous quality improvement (CQI)*.

Even hospitals with the best clinical services may deliver those services inefficiently. Long waits may exist at the emergency room or for admissions. Communications among different clinical departments treating the same patient may not always be clear. Avoidable errors may occur and may be costly to correct.

Under a cost-based reimbursement system, the penalties for inefficiency are not always apparent. Under a prospective payment system, quality improvement will not only result in better care but will also result in more cost-effective care, increasing productivity and efficiency.

Traditional quality assurance in the medical field has involved the screening of charts for adverse occurrences and identifying those occurrences with the responsible physician. Donald M. Berwick, a proponent of CQI, describes this approach to quality assurance—quality assurance by inspection—as the "Theory of Bad Apples."[12] This approach dominates thinking in the health care field and, according to Berwick, has failed American industry for many years. He urges the adoption by the health care industry of principles developed by W. Edwards Deming and Joseph M. Juran in the early 1930s at what is now the AT&T Bell Laboratories. These principles are based on the perception that problems are usually built into the complex production processes that these investigators studied. They concluded that defects in quality could seldom be attributed to a lack of will, skill, or benign intention among the people involved with the processes. Rather than seeking to establish guilt, under their theory organizations should examine the production process to see how it could be improved and the problem eliminated.

There is some doubt about the portability of CQI from industry to the health care field. William R. Fifer, who has had many years of experience with quality in health care, in addition to other concerns, doubts that the health care field as a whole possesses sufficient organizational competence to accomplish the shift of direction from traditional quality assurance methods to CQI.[13] Nevertheless, some hospitals trying CQI programs have had remarkable success. All hospitals should try them.

Improving Board-Staff Relations

Trustees need to be attentive to several aspects of board-staff relations.

Organization of the Medical Staff

Every hospital must have an organized medical staff. The structure, membership, and function of this organization are prescribed by medical staff bylaws, which vary substantially from hospital to hospital. The leadership may include both institutional leadership by officers elected by the medical staff and clinical leadership by department chairs and chiefs of divisions. Clinical leadership may be combined with institutional leadership under a chief of staff designated by the board or elected by the staff.

The medical staff bylaws generally

- Designate the general officers of the medical staff, their method of selection, and their duties.
- Specify classes of staff membership such as active staff, courtesy staff, consulting staff, and emeritus staff, and the prerogatives and obligations of the members of each class.
- Establish qualifications for the extension and delineation of clinical privileges.
- Organize the medical staff into major clinical departments such as medicine or surgery, and within those departments, into appropriate divisions such as (in the department of medicine) cardiology, internal medicine, gastroenterology, and so on. They also describe the administrative and quality assurance functions of each department and division.
- Determine how department chairs and division chiefs are to be chosen, unless this is covered by the corporate bylaws, and delineate their responsibilities.
- Establish an executive committee (required by the JCAHO *Accreditation Manual*[14]) and other standing committees and describe the purposes and composition of each. Such committees, in addition to the executive, might include clinical care, planning, education and research, credentials, and nominating.
- Describe occasions and procedures for disciplining members.
- Prescribe procedures, usually called a *fair hearing plan,* for guaranteeing procedural due process and appellate review rights to staff members in the event of a disciplinary proceeding, denial of or reduction in privileges, or the refusal to grant a request for additional privileges.[15]

Medical staff bylaws are usually developed and periodically revised by a staff bylaws committee, adopted by the full staff, and submitted to the governing board for its approval.

The legal status of medical staff bylaws after their adoption is not clear. There is some case law to the effect that the bylaws constitute a contract between the medical staff and the hospital. "Neither party may unilaterally amend the medical staff bylaws."[16]

The medical staff generally consists of salaried and nonsalaried physicians. Ancillary services in hospitals are frequently provided by full-time salaried physicians, while medical and surgical care is provided by private "attending" physicians, who are compensated by the patient and not the hospital for their services. In recent years, larger teaching hospitals have increasingly employed physicians as department chairs and division chiefs to provide professional and clinical administrative services. These arrangements, on occasion, have caused some dismay on the part of the private attending physicians and are viewed by them as a threat to fee-for-service medicine. Because the salaried physicians usually have distinguished academic backgrounds and a strong interest in research and education, a type of "town-gown" tension can develop between these two groups. A board of trustees that is contemplating moving in the direction of having salaried physicians head any of its clinical divisions should weigh the presumed benefits of the arrangements against the risk of possibly alienating a substantial number of the private attending physicians. A board statement citing benefits of the arrangement may help to alleviate the tensions such an arrangement may cause. These benefits include relief of the attending physicians from burdensome administrative duties, freeing them for full-time fee-for-service medical practice.

The Need for Collegiality

Physicians bring different training, experience, and objectives to bear on hospital problems than do members of the board, whose experience, attitudes, and concerns may also differ from those of the CEO and members of the administrative staff. As to patient care matters, for example, physicians should bring clinical detachment and objectivity to patient care management, while the CEO may be more concerned with operational and fiscal considerations. Trustees should be concerned with all of the above, as well as with the interests of the community. A hospital's success depends on these three groups being able to accommodate each other's varying interests and concerns harmoniously and cordially. This goal can only be accomplished if there is an atmosphere of mutual respect and trust.

In this equation, the physicians are presumptively qualified to deal with hospital issues relating to the delivery of medical care within the institution. They have been licensed to practice medicine, admitted to the organized medical staff, and achieved some success as medical practitioners. By virtue of the CEO's appointment to the position by the members of the governing board after reviewing his or her credentials, the chief executive is presumptively qualified to deal with hospital problems. The unknown part of the equation is the hospital trustees. Although the CEO will usually accept their qualifications on faith, it is the trustees' responsibility to convince the physicians that they understand the problems of the hospital, will contribute materially to their solutions, and deserve the physicians' cooperation and support. Their divergent interests and backgrounds not only create a unique relationship between members of the board and the medical staff but also a delicate one. The board's responsibilities may place members from time to time in opposition to the organized medical staff or some of its members. The institution should see that every effort is made to avoid confrontation and to relieve the tensions such opposition can induce. Some tension between board and medical staff will always exist, but every effort should be made to keep this to a minimum.

One of the major obstacles to board–medical staff rapprochement is that of adequate communication. Physicians may feel frustrated at the difficulty of appropriateness of approaching governing board members directly, particularly in situations where they feel that their interests or concerns have been incompetently or unfairly handled by the administration. Board members may feel uncomfortable in approaching physicians directly, since this could be viewed as undermining the authority of the CEO or the medical staff leadership and as establishing a cumbersome second step for handling problems. But mechanisms should be in place to foster such direct interactions.

The easiest solution is to include medical staff members on the board by having the hospital's bylaws provide for certain staff officers to serve as ex-officio members of the board. But this is not always the best solution. Such representation may be highly formalistic and limited to the delivering of routine medical staff reports by the ex-officio members at regularly scheduled meetings. Also, disaffected physicians, because of medical staff politics, may have no reasonable expectation that the ex-officio medical staff board members will come to their defense.

In addition to board membership by physicians, a variety of other approaches are available to enhance board–medical staff communication. In resolving quality issues, some hospitals have regularly scheduled luncheon meetings for representatives of the medical staff and board executive committee at which such matters can be reviewed.[17] Another approach has been to allow individual physicians to place items on the meeting agenda of the joint conference or medical affairs committee. A third possibility is the creation of a standing committee of the board, designated as the medical staff liaison committee and consisting of no more than three very senior board members who would be readily available to respond to the concerns of disturbed or disaffected members of the medical staff. Whatever the solution, the goal should be to enable medical staff members to constructively ventilate their dissatisfactions without adversely affecting relationships within the institution.

A number of factors influence the success of a hospital, but probably nothing could more favorably influence its success than having the most respected and qualified physicians in the community on its medical staff and being the institution of choice for the hospitalization of their patients. In metropolitan areas, many physicians have multiple staff appointments and have the ability, in many cases, to transfer their principal practice from one institution to another with little difficulty. Therefore, it behooves the hospital board to make sure that the practice of attending patients within its institution is as attractive as possible to its medical staff members.

Credentialing

The credentialing of physicians and the delineation of their privileges is very central to the responsibility of the governing board. The success of the institution and the care and safety of its patients depend on the competence, skill, and diligence of the attending physicians. The board has the responsibility, through the credentialing and recredentialing process, to ensure that all physicians who are accorded staff privileges are qualified to practice in the areas to which their privileges extend and that they exercise those privileges competently and diligently. The board and its individual members should bear in mind the institution's responsibility and liability for the practice of medicine by its physicians under the decision in the *Darling* case.[18]

    Credentialing of physicians and the delineation of their privileges is partially delegated by the board to the medical staff primarily because the medical staff is viewed as being in a better position to adequately assess a physician's capabilities. The role the board plays is largely one of oversight, to make sure that the methods followed by the staff in developing information on candidates for staff privileges are adequate, fair, and accurate and free of legal problems. The ultimate legal responsibility for credentialing, however, rests with the board and cannot be delegated entirely to the medical staff.

    Hospitals may go beyond mere state licensure in their standards for medical staff membership. Additional requirements should reasonably relate to the competence of the physicians and their ability to render high-quality medical care at the institution. These requirements may include specialized training such as board certification or board eligibility in a medical specialty; meaningful experience at other institutions where the physician has had privileges; moral, physical, and ethical fitness to engage in medical practice; and lack of disruptiveness in dealing with medical and administrative personnel. Under certain circumstances, a candidate may also be required to agree to practice primarily at the specific institution. Candidates who are otherwise qualified may be rejected if their office is distant from the hospital, they refuse to carry adequate amounts of medical malpractice insurance, or they hold numerous staff appointments at other hospitals. The section on "Medical Staff Development Plans" later in this chapter suggests some additional bases for rejection.

Legally unacceptable reasons for rejection of qualified candidates include requiring membership in the local medical society, holding a D.O. rather than an M.D. degree, and requiring sponsorship by a current member of the staff. While legal counsel for the hospital review any credentialing provisions in the corporate or medical staff bylaws and evaluate them under antitrust criteria, the individual trustees should be aware of some of the guidelines in the area.

The board has the power under certain circumstances to completely close its staff to new members. Such closure would only seem to be justified when the equipment and facilities of the institution are unable to accommodate patients admitted by any additional staff members. Although closing the staff completely would be unusual, hospitals frequently will, in effect, close an ancillary department such as pathology, anesthesiology, or radiology by contracting with a particular physician or physician group to provide this service on an exclusive basis. These arrangements can often be justified by the increased efficiency with which the department can be operated and coverage scheduled. If this is done in a one-hospital market, however, it may violate the antitrust laws.

The Fair Hearing Plan

An adverse credentialing decision by the board and/or the medical staff generally entitles the practitioner to certain due process rights designed to ensure that such decisions are not arbitrary or capricious but are based on the competence and qualifications of the practitioner. Credentialing decisions that trigger the due process procedures typically include the following: refusing to grant privileges, refusing to grant requested additional privileges, restricting privileges, or terminating privileges. The Health Care Quality Improvement Act of 1986, the JCAHO *Accreditation Manual for Hospitals,* and the Medicare Conditions for Participation for hospitals require that due process procedures be in place.

Due process protections are usually embodied in a fair hearing plan, which is part of the medical staff bylaws. Generally, the *fair hearing plan* requires that the affected physician be given timely and adequate notice of the reasons for the adverse decision as well as the opportunity for a timely hearing, at which the physician has a right to be heard and to hear the negative testimony. To enhance the impartiality of the proceedings, the tribunal should consist of "fair-minded" persons, including an arbitrator who is mutually agreeable to the hospital and the physician, a hearing officer appointed by the hospital, or a committee comprising physicians who are not competitors of the physician and other persons who have no interest in the outcome. Each side should be entitled to have legal counsel, although the use of legal counsel may tend to bog down the proceedings. If the hearing decision is adverse to the physician, he or she should have the right to appeal to the board of the hospital or to a committee to which the board has delegated this responsibility.

Medical Staff Development Plan

Reference has been made to the need for hospitals to have and retain a highly qualified medical staff. As a corollary to this, hospitals also need to attract younger physicians to the medical staff to replace older physicians who may die or retire. Attracting new physicians will only have optimum benefits for the institution, however, if it is done on a selective basis regarding medical specialties and subspecialties.

The objective of retaining a strong medical staff is to have the optimum number of staff physicians in each medical specialty and subspecialty to serve the perceived health needs of the institution's service area. This can be done by adopting a *medical staff development plan* and making an analysis of each practice area within the institution.

Some hospitals may have more practitioners in a particular specialty than the institution can reasonably accommodate. Accordingly, membership in these departments or divisions is often closed to new appointees until attrition has reduced the number of practitioners in that specialty below the optimum or until additional facilities are added. The area will then be reopened for membership until enough additional practitioners have been credentialed to meet the hospital's resources in the specialty.

Where there are insufficient practitioners in a specialized medical practice area to meet the community need, these areas remain open to new staff appointments. Often hospitals will make efforts to recruit new staff members to fill these vacancies.

When a practice area is closed, applications for appointment should only be accepted with the understanding that they will not be acted on until a vacancy occurs. When the vacancy occurs, the applications should be considered and priorities established on the basis of the relative merit of the applicants rather than by giving priority to the time of filing.

Medical Staff Development Funds

Some of the more successful hospitals have established *medical staff development funds* to furnish no-interest or low-interest loans to physicians who may be interested in establishing their practices within the hospital's service area or to otherwise provide financial support to newly recruited physicians.

Entering into such arrangements and making such loans, while desirable, must be done with great care. These arrangements may violate the fraud and abuse provisions of the Medicare and Medicaid laws, jeopardize the hospital's exempt status under the federal tax laws, or violate the antitrust laws. Therefore, the advice of the hospital's legal counsel in entering into such financial arrangements should be sought and carefully followed.

Decisions as to whether a medical staff development plan is adopted or whether a medical staff development fund is established involve institutional policy as determined by the governing board. Implementation of these plans and their monitoring will require expert medical input furnished by either the medical staff or outside medical consultants. Once again, the responsibility for the success or failure of any such plan or related fund lies with the board.

Antitrust and the Health Care Quality Improvement Act of 1986

The failure to grant or the reduction or withdrawal of medical staff privileges by hospitals has been a fertile basis for the filing of antitrust cases by disappointed physicians against (1) the hospitals, (2) the physicians who participated in the credentialing process, and (3) the members of the governing boards. Aggrieved physicians often allege that the adverse decision regarding their privileges amounts to a contract, combination, or conspiracy in restraint of trade under Section 1 of the Sherman Act or an attempt at monopoly power under Section 2. In addition to the potential for large damage awards, these cases are typically protracted, extremely expensive to defend, and involve strong emotional involvement on both sides. One case, *Patrick v. Burgett,* which was decided by the U.S. Supreme Court in 1988, is a good example of the problems in this area.[19] In 1981, Dr. Timothy Patrick sued the hospital and the physicians who had participated in the credentialing proceeding that terminated his medical staff privileges. His complaint alleged violations of Sections 1 and 2 of the Sherman Act and Oregon State Antitrust Law. Despite the defendants' claims that their activities were protected by the state's peer review laws, the jury verdict was against the physician defendants (the hospital settled before trial). Dr. Patrick was awarded $650,000 in damages, which was trebled to $1,950,000, as permitted under the Sherman Act, plus $250,000 in counsel fees. The verdict was reversed on appeal to the 9th Circuit Court of Appeals but reinstated by the Supreme Court. The effect of this lengthy litigation on all of the physicians involved, including Dr. Patrick, was catastrophic. The wide publicity generated in the medical community and the destructive impact on the participants has negatively affected the willingness of some medical staff members to voluntarily participate in hospital credentialing and peer review activities and has handicapped hospitals' efforts to conduct peer review and credentialing.

Following the decision of the lower court in *Patrick,* Representative Ron Wyden of Oregon introduced legislation that was enacted as the *Health Care Quality Improvement Act of 1986* with the purpose of enhancing the peer review process and improving the quality of care.[20] In addition to establishing a national data bank and requiring the reporting of certain adverse actions relating to physician incompetence, the act requires that hospitals request information from the data bank on reported actions when credentialing or recredentialing a physician. The act provides a limited immunity for participants in credentialing and peer review activities if the institution is in compliance with the act; the professional review action was taken in the reasonable belief that it was in furtherance of quality health care; a reasonable effort was made to obtain the facts in the matter; and after adequate notice, fair hearing procedures were afforded to the physician involved. While the protection afforded by the act is tenuous, all hospitals should have their counsel review their corporate and medical staff bylaws as well as the hospital's fair hearing plan to ensure that the hospital is in compliance with the act.

Physicians as Trustees

Should physician members of the medical staff serve on the governing boards of their hospitals? In the past, this has often been answered in the negative because of the belief that physician staff members have a conflict of interest that precludes their being able to discharge their responsibilities as trustees. It is difficult to understand, however, how mere membership on both the medical staff and board would create a disqualifying conflict between the physicians and the institution. Assuming the physicians do not have some special business arrangement with the hospital, membership on the board might appear to give them an opportunity to compete unfairly with other members of the medical staff, but not necessarily with the institution itself. The physicians' staff membership should be a well-known fact to their colleagues on the board. If an item comes before the board in which they have an interest, they should disclose their interest and decline to participate in any discussion or vote with respect to that item. Compliance with Judge Gesell's rules as set forth in the *Sibley* case should eliminate any potential problems.[21]

On the other hand, there are good reasons, in addition to the communications problem previously discussed, why qualified physicians should be accorded board membership. First, without physician membership, the board may not be fully informed of what is going on in the hospital from a medical standpoint. If there is a *medical director,* his or her attendance at board meetings would ameliorate the situation, but often the medical director, merely by holding that position, is distanced from the attending physicians and may not be as well informed as other physicians. A second reason for having physician board members is that it provides an additional source of information from the medical staff about their problems and concerns, which, without contact through board membership, might never get reported.

Perhaps the best reason for having physicians on the governing boards of hospitals has to do with the unique organizational structure of hospitals. In a university setting, the president has an academic background, and in the business world, the CEO has a business background. This is not so in the hospital setting; the hospital chief executive seldom has a medical background. It is important to the hospital that a firsthand source of medical knowledge and experience be an integral part of the board's resources and be included in its deliberations. The only practical way to accomplish this is to have one or more physicians serve as members of the board.[22] There are no compelling reasons why those physicians should not be from the hospital's own medical staff.

Peer Review Organizations

In 1983, the Peer Review Improvement Act[23] replaced professional standards review organizations (PSROs), which had been organized around a regional Health Systems Agency (HSA), with statewide *peer review organizations (PROs)* under contract with the Health Care Finance Administration. State PROs review the hospital care of Medicare patients to determine the necessity, appropriateness, and adequacy of their treatment. All hospitals treating Medicare patients are required to maintain a contract with their state PRO to provide this service. The 1991 budget for the PRO program was $330 million, or 0.3 percent of Medicare expenditures.[24]

CHAPTER 11

Knowing When and How to Restructure

Over the past several years, many hospitals in this country have undergone a process of corporate reorganization that has transformed the traditional single corporation hospital into a multicorporation hospital.[1] Typically, these new hospitals continue to exist as the providers of inpatient care. Other hospital activities, however, are now being transferred to different corporations within the hospital group. The reasons for this corporate reorganization include the following:

- Maximizing reimbursement
- Protecting assets from tort and contract liability
- Avoiding jeopardizing the hospital's tax exempt status by its engaging in substantial taxable activity
- Avoiding the inclusion of non–patient care activities and revenue in the financial audits by state and federal agencies
- Avoiding certificate of need and other hospital-oriented regulatory requirements for non–patient care projects
- Facilitating the acquisition or development of profitable business activities to be used to provide independent income streams to the hospital
- Providing a corporate structure that would facilitate the acquisition, governance, and management of new busi-

nesses, joint ventures, and other endeavors, including projects with other health care providers

The incentive of improving reimbursement, usually by taking unreimbursable cost centers out of the hospital and placing them in nonprovider corporations, is only effective where there is a cost-based reimbursement system. Cost reimbursement has become less significant for most hospitals because of DRGs. Therefore, attempting to maximize reimbursement has become a less compelling reason for restructuring.

Taking major assets, such as endowment, out of the provider corporation may serve to protect these assets from attachment if there is a large tort liability judgment entered against the hospital.

If a tax exempt corporation, like a hospital, engages in an excessive amount of taxable activity, this will jeopardize its exempt status. If this activity is transferred to a taxable corporate affiliate, the activity should not affect the hospital's exemption.

Because compliance with the audit requirements imposed on hospitals by state and federal agencies can be both costly and burdensome, removing all but patient care–related matters from the hospital corporation can substantially reduce such burdens. (This benefit is offset, however, by the added burden of maintaining separate accounting systems for each of the newly created corporations.)

The hospitals may avoid the necessity of a certificate-of-need procedure by having an affiliated corporation undertake a project in place of the hospital. Opportunities for avoidance of certificate of need are not, however, always available. Care should be taken to ensure that the state regulatory authorities agree that the project is not reviewable.

In many cases, the most valuable advantage provided by restructuring is the ability of one of the nonprovider corporations to (1) enter into relationships with alternative delivery systems, (2) enter into joint ventures with physician groups, and (3) network with other hospitals or hospital groups. These beneficial activities might be inhibited or prohibited if such relationships could only be entered into by the hospital corporation.

The creation and operation of these new corporations, some with missions only tangentially related to the delivery of in-house acute health care, generate problems that are foreign to many hospital executives. A hospital executive's specialized education, training, and practical experience in traditional hospital administration are of limited use in determining how a hospital should now interrelate with its affiliates.

Among units of a multiform corporate structure, the division of functions that were previously performed by a single corporation creates problems of organization and communication and places additional burdens on governing boards and management teams alike. The alleviation of these problems in many ways is more a matter of governance than of management. Trustee input is needed.

In the typical restructuring, a "parent" corporation is created. To become a parent corporation of a for-profit subsidiary, the parent acquires the shares of the subsidiary. To become the subsidiary of a parent nonprofit corporation, a nonprofit corporation amends its bylaws to cede to the parent corporation one or more of the following functions of government: (1) to name the members of its board, (2) to approve any changes in its charter or bylaws, (3) to approve any borrowings it may make, and (4) to approve its long-range strategic plan and capital and operating budgets.

Figure 1 shows a diagram of a simple restructured hospital corporation.

Board Composition and Committee Structure

The first task confronting the restructured hospital is to determine which members of the hospital board will continue as hospital board members, which members will govern the other corporations in the system, and which members will have overlapping board memberships. Although it is helpful

Figure 1. A Simple Restructured Hospital Corporation.

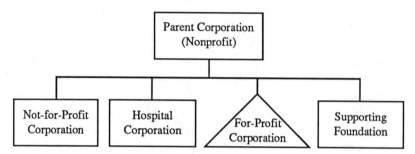

to have some overlapping board memberships, members of the hospital board should not constitute a majority of the membership of the parent corporation board in order to avoid the appearance that the hospital, in fact, controls the parent.

The reassignment of board members can best be accomplished if the board chair first discusses the matter with the board members to get their views and preferences as to their assignments.

The next problem is to establish the committee structure for the parent corporation. In doing this, there should be a clear understanding of the parent corporation's role and mission. The parent corporation should have its own mission statement and long-range strategic plan. These plans should take into account that the role of the parent corporation is to provide coordination and direction for the system. This involves selecting (and, if necessary, removing) members of the governing boards of the affiliates, allocating the assets of the affiliates, and developing long-range plans for the system. Implicit in the responsibilities of the parent corporation is the evaluation of individual governing boards of the affiliates.

The Need for Maintaining Separate Entities

Not only must hospitals form separate legal entities to realize the benefits of restructuring, but they must also design a structure to allow these separate entities to operate in such a way that the courts and the state and federal regulatory agencies will regard them as having a separate legal existence. Systems must not operate in a fashion that blurs the corporate distinctions. This might allow a court or regulatory agency to "pierce the corporate veil" and determine that any two or more of these separate corporations actually represent a single legal and economic entity.

Courts, in determining whether or not to ignore the separate existence of related corporations and to treat them as a single entity, have given consideration to the following factors:

- The parent company's ownership of all or a majority of the capital stock of the subsidiary
- The presence of common officers and directors
- The failure to observe corporate formalities, such as separate board and shareholder meetings and keeping separate corporate minutes
- The nature of the transactions between the parent company and the subsidiary
- The degree of intervention of the parent company into the financial activities, business, and affairs of the subsidiary
- Holding the subsidiary out to the public as a department or division of the parent company
- The undercapitalization of the subsidiary

Generally speaking, the presence of one or more of these elements does not settle the issue of separate corporate existence. The courts will examine the totality of the circumstances before deciding whether or not to collapse the corporations into each other. Conversely, where the subsidiary carefully maintains its separate existence, the courts generally will not collapse the corporations despite the fact that some of the factors noted above may be present.

The hazards in failing to maintain the separateness of the corporations in the restructured system might include loss of tax exemption, a corporation in the system being held liable for the obligations incurred by or imposed on another corporation in the system, the necessity of obtaining a certificate of need when this would otherwise not have been necessary, and the possibility that income from an otherwise separate freestanding support foundation would be used to reduce the hospital's rate base in a rate-regulation state.

Observing the following should reduce the risk of the involuntary collapse of the separate corporations in the system into each other:

- The overlap between boards should be less than half and preferably no more than one-third of the total.
- Boards of the corporations should meet separately and regularly. (It is generally recommended that a board meet no less often than once a year.)
- The committee structure of the parent corporation should relate to its mission and should not parallel the committee structure of the hospital.
- All business transactions between the corporations should be at arm's length. Transfers of funds from one of the corporations to another should be documented and supported by a written record of board action.

As has been previously pointed out, operating a restructured hospital is much more burdensome than operating a single corporation hospital. Administration must arrange, provide staffing, and attend many more corporate board and committee meetings. The fiscal officers must also maintain separate sets of books. In addition, meetings are often repetitious, in view of the usual requirement that the parent approve all transactions except for those transactions that are in the ordinary course of business of the subsidiaries. And there is a strong temptation to have joint committee meetings, have the hospital and holding company boards meet together, and have the hospital's board action and the holding company's board approval take place at the same time.

The configuration of the restructured corporations

should be reviewed each year as part of the board's self-evaluation. The structure should be fine-tuned and reduced to the simplest form that will accomplish its goals. At that time, the board should also consider whether it is worth the extra effort to operate in a restructured configuration. If it determines that it is not, the restructured organization should be returned to its original form.

The Restructuring Backlash

Municipalities having difficulty finding the funds with which to pay for municipal services have begun to look askance at hospitals and the exemption from real estate taxes they enjoy. This is an exemption as old as the hospitals themselves. The almshouses and early hospitals, in serving the poor, were models of charitable endeavor. Tax assessors looking at restructured hospitals today, however, see organizations that seem to allocate very little of their assets to the relief of the poor. In fact, those restructured hospitals with holding companies and affiliates engaged in for-profit businesses appear to the taxing authorities much more like present-day commercial or industrial enterprises than the shelters for the ill and impoverished that their founders had established.

Challenges have been made to real estate tax exemption for certain hospitals, and eventually these cases have come to the courts. While a number of these cases were decided in favor of the institutions, certain significant cases were not. Some of the courts thought that the hospitals had, in the restructuring process, abandoned their public service missions and were utilizing assets originally dedicated to charity for commercial purposes in competition with local tax-paying entities. As mentioned in Chapter Four, in a Pennsylvania decision, the Court of Common Pleas of Erie County, Pennsylvania, held, after an examination of Hamot Medical Center's corporate structure and activities, that Hamot's primary purpose was no longer charitable.[2]

Hamot Medical Center, a large and successful hospital, had been founded in 1881 and restructured in 1981. It then

became part of a twenty-corporation system under Hamot
Health System, Inc. (HHSI). Between 1981 and 1989, when
this proceeding was instituted, the hospital transferred $25
million to HHSI and to Hamot Corporate Services, Inc.,
which provided management and administrative services for
the affiliated corporations. These funds were used to purchase
property and establish various businesses, including a marina,
a pharmacy, a health club, a retirement center, and an office
building, in competition with local enterprises. No funds
were returned to Hamot Medical Center for health care purposes. The court determined that the promotion of health
was no longer Hamot's primary purpose and that all property, including that of the hospital, was subject to real estate
taxation. The court noted that if the Hamot Corporate Services structure should change, it would consider modifying
its order.

A growing dissatisfaction with the operating problems
of restructured hospitals and judicial decisions like *Hamot*[3]
have resulted in many restructured hospitals spinning off
their for-profit enterprises, particularly those not integral to
the hospital mission. CEOs of hospitals having several subsidiary operating businesses, many of them little more than
marginal "mom and pop" operations, found themselves
expending major amounts of time and energy trying to make
these businesses profitable. This was time taken away from
the hospital, which needed full-time attention.

CHAPTER 12

The Impact of Shared Services and Managed Care

In this chapter, we take up shared services as well as managed care systems such as HMOs and PPOs.

Federal Encouragement of Multihospital Systems

During the past twenty years, the investor-owned hospital chains have enjoyed spectacular success. As large, multi-institutional enterprises, they were apparently able to develop economies of scale not available to most freestanding not-for-profit hospitals. In the National Health Planning and Resources Development Act of 1974, Congress established, among other things, three national health care priorities:[1]

1. The development of "multi-institutional systems for the coordination or consolidation of institutional health services"[2]
2. The creation of "multi-institutional arrangements for the sharing of (hospital) support services"[3]
3. The capacity to provide health care "on a geographically integrated basis"[4]

Congress apparently felt that the development of multi-institutional facilities would tend to eliminate duplication of services, provide economies of scale, and result in a more rationally developed national health care delivery system.

Religious Sponsorship and University Affiliation

Among nonprofit hospitals, those established by a religious organization are frequently united under common ownership and control. Few university hospitals are under common ownership and control with the university except for heavily endowed institutions like Johns Hopkins, state-aided institutions like the University of Pennsylvania, and large land-grant colleges such as those in Michigan, Texas, Missouri, Colorado, Iowa, and Kansas.[5]

One of the recommendations of the *Flexner Report,* as previously noted, was that medical schools should be linked with hospitals. This led to a movement toward medical school–hospital affiliation. Such affiliations were accomplished by the parties entering into an affiliation agreement that usually provided that appointments to the medical staffs of the member hospitals were to originate in the faculty of the school of medicine. They also provided that the chairs of the various clinical departments at the medical school were to serve as chairs of the same clinical departments of the hospital. These affiliation agreements nearly always make it possible for staff members of affiliated hospitals to have staff privileges, as appropriate, at other affiliated hospitals and to be members of the faculty of the medical school.

Other Systems

A study of multi-institutional health care systems[6] examined a number of these organizations. They reflected varying institutional interrelationships, including the following:

> Hospitals affiliated through common management under contract
> Hospitals affiliated through the provision of shared clinical services

Hospitals having separate clinical facilities affiliated through statutory consolidation or merger

Hospitals affiliated by a large urban hospital providing resources to permit the development of a regional health care system of smaller hospitals

Hospitals affiliated by a centrally located hospital developing satellite facilities in other parts of its statewide service area

Alliances

Hospitals have entered into several other types of affiliations. One example is the type of national alliance or hospital consortium represented by Voluntary Hospitals of America (VHA), which has 664 member hospitals representing 208,823 beds and operates twenty-nine regional health care systems.[7] There are other national alliances like American Health Care Systems and regional alliances such as Pacific Health Alliance, alliances of specialized hospitals, and alliances of hospitals sponsored by church or other religious groups.

The purpose of an alliance is to try to give its members many of the benefits of being part of a large multihospital system while continuing to exist as freestanding, self-governing, voluntary institutions. Alliance members are selected from among hospitals that do not directly compete with each other and that are organized largely on a state-by-state basis. At regular state meetings, members discuss their current operations and prospective plans in order to develop mutually supportive programs to increase their market shares and revenues. At the national level, VHA provides purchasing and financial services that the individual members would be unable to obtain independently. Additional services and programs are also available to the members if they wish to subscribe. Members may display a VHA logo and participate in a joint advertising program. Efforts by VHA to develop managed care and other programs in connection with a large insurance company have, so far, met with indifferent success.

It is important for hospital board members to be aware

of the almost limitless variety of arrangements that a hospital may make with other health care institutions. This awareness enables hospital board members to understand and work with management to effect arrangements that will permit the hospital to accomplish results it could not accomplish alone.

According to *Trustee* magazine, alliances experienced a growth rate of 250 percent between 1984 and 1986.[8] It is obvious that alliance memberships are beneficial to many hospitals. Alden T. Solovy notes in the article just cited that hospitals should shop for an alliance and find one whose programs are consonant with the hospital's business plan, whose members are compatible, and who share the same philosophy as the shopping institution.

Gerald L. McManis, a Washington, D.C., management consultant, believes that many alliances have erred in offering too many support services without fully developing and refining any of them.[9] He believes that alliances must provide an otherwise indispensable service to their members and focus on value.

HMOs

In an effort to effect economies of scale and to provide quality health care at a reduced cost to large corporate employee and other subscriber groups, various types of alternative delivery systems have developed over the past several years that have had a substantial impact on the economics of health care delivery. More than 60,000,000 Americans have health coverage through HMOs and PPOs.[10]

Although alternative delivery systems take various forms, all of them contract for reduced rates with the hospitals they utilize. Further, these alternative delivery systems provide effective preadmission and concurrent utilization review and require second opinions on all surgery.

HMOs have developed as a means of providing health care to substantial identifiable groups of subscribers with the expectation that the cost will be less than if conventional delivery mechanisms had been used. They are favored by large-employer purchasers of health care as enabling them to purchase on a wholesale rather than a retail basis. An HMO offers a broad range of health care services, including physician care and hospitalization.

In the *staff* model HMO, the subscriber-patient is seen at the HMO's facilities by a physician employed by the HMO.

In the *group* plan, a group of physicians contract with the HMO to provide medical care for its subscribers.

In the *independent practice association (IPA)* model, individual physicians enter into contracts with the HMO and patients are seen in the physician's private offices.

Hospitalization is at a hospital designated by the HMO. Subscribers pay a flat per capita fee for the services they receive. The HMO bears the economic risk of a member having a long and costly illness. Irrespective of cost of health care to an individual subscriber, the subscription fee for that subscriber remains the same.

Because the HMO is at risk for the cost of care and has mechanisms for screening out unnecessary care, it must also determine whether the care provided is adequate to ensure subscriber satisfaction. HMOs must prevent the erosion of their own marketplace.

The HMO provides exclusive service in the sense that the subscriber is obligated to use the HMO's facilities and health care practitioners. This is in contrast to a traditional insurance plan offered by Blue Cross that pays a negotiated rate to the hospital chosen by the subscriber. Likewise, Blue Shield will pay the usual and customary fee for services of the physician of the subscriber's choice.

PPOs

PPOs provide health care to subscribers through physicians and health care institutions with which the PPO has entered into preferred provider arrangements. These preferred provider arrangements usually call for reimbursement at a discount from hospital charges and from usual and customary charges for physicians. PPOs will ordinarily pay for services from other physicians and institutions but in an amount less than they will pay if their member physicians and institutions are utilized. The reductions usually take the form of increased deductibles or copayments by the patient. A PPO is not an insurer and its charges to subscribers are directly related to the services provided.

HMOs, PPOs, and the Hospital

HMOs are subject to regulation by certain federal statutes and, because of their risk assumption as to the cost of health care to their subscribers, they are regulated by most state insurance commissions. PPOs arguably do not have such risks and are subject to less regulation.

HMOs, as was previously pointed out, are paid a flat charge per member. PPOs have, with each institution with which they contract, a negotiated per diem rate, per case rate, or a fixed reduction in rate from normal charges. Generally, PPOs also have a negotiated rate for services to be provided by the physicians with whom they contract.

In many hospitals, members of the medical staff have formed organizations to represent the member physicians in the negotiation of physician fee contracts with alternative provider organizations. These negotiating organizations generally exist separate from the hospital medical staff organization.

The success of PPOs is thought to be less dependent on their ability to negotiate reduced fees than on their ability to prevent their subscribers from receiving unnecessary or inappropriate care. Rigorous utilization review and the use of second opinions in surgical cases have had this effect.

In addition, the "gatekeeper system" has been very effective in reducing hospitalization by alternative delivery system subscribers. Under this system, every subscriber has a primary care (gatekeeper) physician. This physician is paid a flat amount per patient per year. No recommendation may be made that the patient see a specialist or be hospitalized except by the primary care physician. Each hospitalization or referral of a patient to a specialist for treatment reduces the amount the primary care physician will be paid for the care of that patient for that year.

The gatekeeper under such a system has a clear conflict of interest, which leads to the following question: If the alternative delivery system does not reveal this conflict of interest to its subscribers, as a matter of policy should the hospital require that it be revealed as a condition of providing services?

It is generally desirable for hospitals, where they are offered the opportunity, to enter into contracts to provide services to subscribers of alternative delivery organizations on a nonexclusive basis. This should increase the hospital's census and provide it with paying patients. The downside of the equation is that these patients' hospital care will be paid for at a rate less than hospital charges. This is usually a minor consideration, however, since very few users pay full charges.

The board should adopt certain minimal standards for its dealings with all alternative delivery systems. These minimal standards should include the following: requiring these organizations to meet certain levels of medical competency, agreeing on a range of discount from charges or other payment arrangements to be offered, obtaining assurances as to the economic viability of the HMO or PPO, and reviewing the HMO's or PPO's record for timely payment and its policies on utilization review. The board should also be concerned about the expectations of the medical staff regarding what practice enhancement opportunities these arrangements will make available to them, including the establishment of a fair fee schedule.

Future Trends

Although HMOs and PPOs have not proven to be effective cost-containment mechanisms, it is expected that by the year 2000, 90 percent of health care will be delivered through managed care organizations.

From its inception, managed care has continually evolved. As this development continues, the distinctions between HMOs and PPOs will blur. Other types of managed care organizations will appear, such as *total managed care organizations (TCMOs).* These will manage all of an employer's health care expenditures, including workers' compensation and the costs associated with the lost time and low productivity of disabled workers.

Developing medical technology and the ability of computer-based information systems to track the outcome of medical treatment may result in the adoption of standardized protocols for health care delivery.

There will be increased direct contracting between large employers and health care delivery systems, including hospitals and multidiscipline physician practice groups.

Although managed care systems today are largely controlled by insurance companies, it is expected that during the next several years, control will pass to physician groups and other providers.[11]

CHAPTER 13

Meeting the Challenge
and Building Effective Boards

When almshouses were evolving into hospitals, hospital governing boards had a close, even intrusive relationship with their institutions. As hospitals became larger and more complex, their operation was turned over to the skilled executives who had been trained to operate them. At the same time, trustees, who were selected for their community influence or financial contributions, failed to keep up with the increasing complexity of their institutions and gradually abdicated their governance functions except with respect to fiscal matters. Hospital boards have simply not, in modern times, been very active or influential in setting the strategic direction of their hospitals. Instead, these boards have been perceived as preservers of the status quo and not as agents of change.[1] The situation is still very much as it was at the beginning of the twentieth century: "Hospital boards met comfortably, month-by-month, with a familiar, self-perpetuating, often self-satisfied cast of characters, whose very presence signified public virtue and social stability."[2] In today's health care crisis, public virtue and social stability are simply not enough. Trustees must be prepared to meet head on the problems facing our health care system and their institutions, to advocate solutions to the problems, and to implement those solutions.

Trustee Responsibility for the System

Boards must provide leadership and direction, not only to their own institutions, but collectively to the entire health care delivery system. To further quote Rosemary Stevens, "Trustees are under special strain. Hospitals may have a future as exemplary social institutions; that is, as institutions where science and humanitarianism, business and ideals are mixed. But trustees have traditionally been conservative (and often uninformed). How far will they wish to (or be able to) define community goals and roles for hospitals? How much influence will they exert? How far will they regain some of the power lost early in the century to doctors and more recently to managers?"[3] All of these are open questions whose resolution will substantially influence the way our health care delivery system works. In essence, Stevens is questioning whether hospital trustees will be part of the problem or part of its solution.

Some observers see trustees emerging as the "rationers of hospital care on behalf of the community" and as the only component of the hospital community "able to achieve a reconciliation of the conflicting demands in a relatively objective manner."[4]

To the extent of their ability and regardless of any obstacles, trustees should become active participants in the resolution of the present crisis. They should support measures that will make health care accessible to the uninsured and the underinsured, that will slow the rise in health care costs, and that will guarantee the delivery of quality health care to all in need without regard to the ability to pay. All of the major health care reform plans that have been developed, some of which are discussed in Chapter One, offer the theoretical capability of accomplishing these goals.

Unfortunately, there are institutional, political, and even legal obstacles to the leadership role of hospital trustees in guiding national health policy in this country.

While the AHA, with the support of the various state associations, has been a leader in establishing national policy for American hospitals, the AHA and the state associations have always been the domain of the hospital CEOs to the virtual exclusion of the hospital trustees. Recently, the AHA has made some efforts to incorporate trustee representation in its policy-making functions. The Congress of Hospital Trustees (the "Congress"), the AHA's forum for trustee activities, consists of trustees representing the various states and a number of trustees at large. While this is a representative trustee group, it is very much a creature of the AHA, controlled as to its activities by the AHA staff assigned to it and the budget allotted to it (without trustee input). In its present form, the Congress will not have an appreciable influence on the AHA. In fact, the existence of the Congress as a separate organization probably is a factor in keeping trustee influence compartmentalized outside the mainstream of AHA activity. Until trustees have a chance to fully participate in the development of policies formulated by the AHA for its member hospitals, it is doubtful that those policies will represent the public interest as fully and fairly as might otherwise be the case. At a time when our health care delivery system needs a complete overhaul, hospital trustees have little opportunity for input into the formulation of the policy that will shape that overhaul.

The inclusion of trustees in policy development would not only ensure a broader and more community-oriented perspective in policy development, but it would increase the likelihood of legislative support and thus the successful implementation of the policies proposed. Trustees are generally perceived to have a more balanced point of view, representing concerns for many different interests, as compared to the relatively narrow interests of the hospital professional. The CEOs, within the framework of the AHA, have done a good job. They are balanced and professional and are an extraordinarily competent group of people. They have been compassionate. But the fact remains that a better job would have been done if the trustees of our community hospitals had been equal participants with them in designing solutions to the problems.

The politicians, in whose hands the ultimate solutions to these problems lie, can be expected to take the politically safe course of least resistance. After implementing only those minimal steps that are absolutely necessary to meet the crisis of the moment, they will likely retreat from the health care arena, leaving for yet another day the fundamental problems that continue to plague our institutions. Trustees should try to prevent this from happening by being stronger advocates at the political level.

Of the problems listed in Chapter One as being responsible for the present crisis, the ones that should be responsive to some form of intervention at the political level include duplication of competitive hospital services, discounts, cost shifting, excessive administrative costs, and excessive malpractice insurance premiums and other costs.

Excess hospital capacity is excluded from the list. It is a problem that can and should be resolved by the hospital community itself without the need for outside intervention. Trustees should lead the way.

It is difficult, however, for trustees to deal directly with each other on the problem of duplication of competitive hospital services because of the antitrust laws. For example, agreements among hospitals concerning which services they will and will not offer are not likely to be viewed favorably under the antitrust laws. For this reason, trustees should work for some accommodation with the Department of Justice to permit consolidation of facilities and services or other arrangements that would produce the sort of cost benefit the antitrust laws were designed to foster.

The problems of discounts and cost shifting will disappear with the adoption of an equitable and predictable reimbursement system that insists on all payers being treated equally.

Excessive administrative and malpractice costs are probably the last two problems that Congress will care to deal with. An attack on either will call forth a redoubtable champion. A critical examination of administrative costs will be considered as a threat, which indeed it is, to the health insurance industry. Any consideration of malpractice and the reform of the tort system for compensating victims of malpractice will bring out the plaintiff's malpractice bar ready to do battle. Congress, still shaken by public response to its catastrophic health coverage initiatives, is not likely, gratuitously, to tackle two old grizzly bears like the insurance industry and the plaintiff's bar at one time. Irrespective of the merits of the arguments of the insurers or those of the lawyers, there are ways administrative costs of providing health care can be very substantially reduced and there are far better ways of resolving malpractice issues than trial by battle, as happens under the present tort system. We must convince Congress of the importance of resolving these issues favorably.

Advocacy

Trustees must communicate their hospitals' needs and their opinions and suggestions to government leaders. Hospital trustees are well suited to this task, since many trustees are familiar with the political process, possess political and community contacts, and, in presenting hospital concerns, take a broad community perspective that makes them credible advocates. Associations, in their public positions on issues, unfortunately, often have a tendency toward overstatement that adversely affects their credibility. To many, such associations are always "crying wolf."

Advocacy does not occur until a policy has been developed and legislative or regulatory action is sought. Trustees should be aware of the policies advocated by hospital associations and the key legislative and regulatory issues affecting their institutions. They should also be aware that policy development at the association level is a complex process, which usually represents a consensus rather than unanimity on the part of the association members.[5]

A variety of forums exist at the national and state level to assist trustees in their advocacy function. The AHA's Congress of Hospital Trustees, previously referred to, provides information to trustees in the form of educational conferences, books, monographs, and a monthly magazine, *Trustee.* It also provides some opportunities for networking that enable trustees from around the country to share and learn from each other.

The Volunteer Trustees of Not-for-Profit Hospitals is a Washington, D.C.-based, 130 plus–member (hospital) organization. It is restricted to not-for-profit hospitals and is primarily focused on federal legislative issues. The organization, through its dedicated and knowledgeable staff, also provides its members with very good and timely information on health care issues and conducts trustee conferences and an annual meeting of its members.

The National Conference of Community Hospitals (NCCH) is another Washington, D.C.-based organization consisting of about 165 community hospitals. This successful advocacy organization is not restricted to trustees and offers timely information and frequent forums for hospital representatives to discuss issues and concerns with federal officials.

Trustees whose hospitals are members of alliances and networks should look for advocacy opportunities available through such affiliations. For example, hospitals with religious affiliations have opportunities for trustee involvement at the national level, through such organizations as the American Protestant Health Association and the Catholic Health Association, the two major national organizations for hospitals with religious affiliations.

There are national organizations for the development of policy and advocacy of issues of particular interest to osteopathic, proprietary, teaching, and various other specialty hospitals. Such organizations include the following:

> American Osteopathic Hospital Association (Alexandria, Virginia)
> Association of American Medical Colleges/Council of Teaching Hospitals (Washington, D.C.)
> Federation of American Health Systems (Washington, D.C.)

National Association of Children's Hospitals and
Related Institutions, Inc. (Alexandria, Virginia)
National Association of Private Psychiatric Hospitals
(Washington, D.C.)
National Association of Rehabilitation Facilities (Washington, D.C.)

At the state level, some state hospital associations have
formed trustee organizations as semi-independent groups to
permit trustee involvement in their associations and as an
effort to meet the educational and informational needs of
trustees. These organizations merit your support and involvement. Their proximity and familiarity with local issues provide a convenient and beneficial means of remaining current
with legislative and regulatory concerns at the state and
national levels.

My own state association, the Hospital Association of
Pennsylvania (HAP), coordinates meetings of trustees with
members of Congress or their staff representatives at the
annual AHA membership meeting in Washington, D.C. This
activity has been well received by trustees and the politicians.
Meetings are scheduled for forty-five minutes. A group of no
more than five trustees will meet for lunch beforehand, preferably in the cafeteria of the Rayburn Office Building, to
determine what message they wish to get across in their meetings with the representatives or their staffs. Although the late
Senator John Heinz always met us in person and participated
in our discussions, some members of Congress prefer to have
their staff members attend the meetings instead. The staff
members are invariably knowledgeable, interested, and determined to understand the concerns of the hospital trustees. I
have always felt that the exchanges of views at these congressional meetings were very useful and that our elected representatives are interested in what trustees have to say.

Another very useful HAP activity is an annual trustee-congressional luncheon held in a hearing room in the Rayburn Building. The luncheon is informal and unstructured,
and careful planning of seating arrangements ensures that

trustees are seated with the senators and representatives they know. Nearly all of the elected delegates attend.

These meetings and luncheons represent advocacy in its most effective forms.

Not all advocacy occurs at the national or state level. Advocacy in health care is to a large extent dictated by public opinion. Hospitals have, in the past, enjoyed the public's support, confidence, and trust. Public opinion trends, however, signify a serious dilemma for leaders of our hospitals. Since the mid 1960s, public confidence in the leaders of medicine and health care institutions has fallen dramatically. This decline is part of a broader trend of growing cynicism toward all major institutions in American society and the growing movement toward commercialization of health care. Trustees must play an important role in renewing public confidence in their institutions and in our health care system generally. Trustees are uniquely situated to explain to their friends, neighbors, business associates, and other community leaders that a well-managed hospital is not managed *for* business principles but *by* business principles. Hospital trustees must build public confidence in order for their institutions to prosper and continue to meet the health care needs of their communities. Hospital trustees, along with other members of the health care team, must become more effective advocates for the patients they expect to serve.

Trustee Responsibility for the Individual Hospital

While trustees have a responsibility for the health care system as a whole, their ultimate legal and moral responsibility is to the individual hospital on whose board they serve.

The changes in the system contemplated by the types of health care reform plans reviewed in Chapter One should benefit all health care institutions. But different reform plans will have different strategic effects on different hospitals. These effects will, among other things, depend on the hospital's location—center city, suburban, or rural; its case mix; its range of services, from primary to tertiary care; its amount of uncompensated care; and other variables.

Coddington, Keen, Moore, and Clarke suggest four possible future scenarios with respect to reform:

Scenario 1: Incremental Changes

- There is continued fragmentation among players.
- Medicare and Medicaid reimbursement does not improve.
- The number of uninsureds increases.
- Competition among hospitals and physician groups grows.
- Duplication of hospital and physician services increases.

Scenario 2: Universal Access/Shakeout of Managed Care

- The number of managed care companies is reduced by half or more.
- There is more market power among payers.
- Employer-based health plans continue.
- Medicare reimbursement is stabilized.

Scenario 3: Universal Access/Consumer Choice

- Consumers purchase health care directly from insurers or managed care firms.
- Incentives are available for consumers to become cost-effective users of the health care system.
- Medicare participants use vouchers to purchase their own health plans.
- Employers may assist employees in purchasing health care but are not of the payment system.

Scenario 4: Universal Access/Single-Payer System

- Either the state or the federal government is the single payer.
- The system is likely to be modeled on the Canadian system.
- Competition among hospitals and physicians diminishes.
- Health plan and insurance industries cease to exist; the need for Medicare disappears.[6]

Scenario 1 is basically a continuation of existing conditions. The other three scenarios, however, represent substantial changes in reimbursement and the other rules of the game. On the premise that no two hospitals are the same or have the same mix of characteristics that would be affected by the type of health care reform adopted, Coddington, Keen, Moore, and Clarke describe the effects of these scenarios on different types of hospitals and suggest strategies that could be adopted in each case. Each individual hospital should, however, analyze its own strengths and weaknesses under these scenarios to determine what steps are best for it. Coddington, Keen, Moore, and Clarke suggest such disparate strategies, under certain circumstances, as primary physician recruitment (always a good one), establishment of a satellite facility at another location, establishment of a tertiary care center of excellence, or development of a nonadversarial relationship with a major health plan. While health care reform is still in the discussion stages, now is the time to prepare for its advent.

Governance in the Future

Except for institutions in such metropolitan areas as San Francisco and New York, no one seems to know what the impact of acquired immune deficiency syndrome (AIDS) will be on our health care institutions during the next several years. Selectively, AIDS will severely impact hospitals in neighborhoods where drug use is the heaviest and whose emergency rooms are already strained by the influx of people afflicted by substance abuse. AIDS will ultimately impact most, if not all, of our hospitals, and we should be developing comprehensive plans to deal with it.

Problematical as the impact of AIDS may be, the problems of an aging population will have greater impact and longer-term implications for our hospital system. Trustees should be preparing to deal with the special needs of this growing segment of their community.

Changing legal limitations on abortion will require

board scrutiny to ensure that the hospital is operating within the legal limits. In addition, trustees must consider the legal and ethical implications of surrogate motherhood, genetic screening, and the withdrawal of life-sustaining treatment. These are areas in which the governing boards, working with community representatives, should provide institutional guidance.

Each year since the Medicare Prospective Payment System went into effect, fewer hospitals have been able to develop positive operating margins. Those with substantial endowments may be able to continue operating at a loss for years to come. Other less fortunate hospitals may soon face bankruptcy or the tougher decisions about primary services and facilities. If your hospital is in one of these categories, is there anything that your board can do by way of an innovative plan to make your institution viable as a hospital? If not, is there another purpose serving the public interest to which the facilities could be put?

Governance is an art, not a science. Primarily, that art involves working with people—fellow board members, administrative officers, physicians, nursing staff, legal counsel, and others who make up the hospital's working family. It also includes relating to people in the community who utilize the hospital and those who support it with their contributions and volunteer efforts. While the trustees and the other members of the hospital's constituency want the same thing for the hospital—for it to become the best it can be—each member of the hospital family will probably have a somewhat different perception of what being the best means and how this common goal can be achieved. Part of an individual trustee's responsibility is to try to bring these divergent perceptions into harmony.

If the national health care delivery system is in need of an overhaul, the same is no less true of the organizational structure of our individual hospitals. As managed care becomes more the rule than the exception, will major corporate employers be willing to take the time and effort to negotiate separate fee arrangements with a hospital and individual members of its medical staff when they can obtain a per diem unit price per patient day from a hospital operated in conjunction with a multidisciplinary physician group? Hospital boards should try to facilitate hospital–medical staff cooperation in the development of organizational structures that offer a unitized service to purchasers of hospital/medical care.

A trustee must be well informed. There is always much to be learned about the science of medicine, the art of healing, and the humanity of caring for others. The learning process also includes the fundamentals of how the hospital can support the efforts of the health care practitioners who provide the medical care and treatment. The learning process is unstructured but continuous.

A good trustee is a good listener. Hospital problems are often complex and cannot be solved unless they are understood. Unfortunately, many hospital problems do not lend themselves to an immediate solution. Other problems may offer several different but equally attractive solutions; the trustee must make the often difficult choice among them.

A trustee who is diligent in attending committee and board meetings, who develops a knowledge of his or her institution, and who works to favorably influence health care policy without regard for institutional or geographical limitations advances the cause of the hospital and provides the community with an institution that better serves its health care needs. This trustee will realize a sense of satisfaction that can rarely be achieved in other public service.

Notes

Chapter One

1. D. Coddington, D. Keen, K. Moore, and R. Clarke, *The Crisis in Health Care: Costs, Choices, and Strategies* (San Francisco: Jossey-Bass, 1990), p. 30.
2. J. Wennberg, J. Freeman, and W. Culp, "Are Hospital Services Rationed in New Haven or Over-Utilized in Boston?," *Lancet*, 1987, 7, 1185.
3. Coddington, Keen, Moore, and Clarke, *The Crisis in Health Care*, p. 21.
4. Coddington, Keen, Moore, and Clarke, *The Crisis in Health Care*, p. 6.
5. Coddington, Keen, Moore, and Clarke, *The Crisis in Health Care*, pp. 120–121.
6. Woolhauphee, S., and Himmelstein, D., "The Deteriorating Administrative Efficiency of the U.S. Health Care System," *New England Journal of Medicine*, May 2, 1991, pp. 1253–1258.
7. Public Citizens Health Records Group, "The Administrative Cost of Health Insurance," *Health Letter*, June 1991, pp. 1–3.
8. Danzon, P. M., " 'The Crisis' in Medical Malpractice: A Comparison of Trends in the United States, Canada, the

United Kingdom, and Australia," *Law, Medicine, &
Health Care,* 1990, *18* (1-2), 48, 54.

Chapter Two

1. Except for relatively minor bureaucratic differences, IBM
   and the Catholic Church bear strong structural similarities to the legions of Imperial Rome. All are pyramidal-
   hierarchical structures.
2. There has never been much uniformity in hospital managerial titles. Originally hospital managers were called
   superintendents. Later this became administrator and,
   in some cases, executive director. Corporate titles for
   management, such as president, vice president, or assis-
   tant vice president, have become popular in the past ten
   years.
3. See F. H. Kerr, "If Boards Mean Business, They'll Refo-
   cus the Governance Function," *Trustee,* Apr. 1983, p. 29.
4. American Hospital Association Resource Center, *Hospital Administration Terminology,* 2nd ed. (Chicago: American Hospital Publishing, 1986), p. 27.
5. See *Hospital Administration Terminology,* pp. 120–121,
   for further discussion of these hospital classifications.
6. *World Almanac and Book of Facts* (1989), p. 814.
7. A note on the term *trustee* may be helpful. Modern nonprofit corporation statutes and the Revised Model Nonprofit Corporation statute of the American Bar Association uniformly designate the members of nonprofit
   corporation governing boards as *directors.* Nonetheless,
   most hospitals seem to have clung to the traditional designation of *trustee.* As so used, the terms are inter-
   changeable.
8. *World Almanac and Book of Facts* (1989), p. 814.
9. Simply stated, the locality rule required that physicians
   in general practice be held to the professional standards
   prevailing in the locality where they practiced rather
   than to a higher national standard. This meant that
   expert testimony regarding medical malpractice had to

come from local physicians, who were often colleagues of the defendant physician and reluctant to testify.

10. J. Califano, "Billions Blown on Health," *New York Times,* Apr. 12, 1989, p. A25.

11. C. E. Rosenberg, *The Care of Strangers* (New York: Basic Books, 1987), p. 116.

12. That a prospect for admission was in need of hospitalization was a given. The committee determined that the prospect was worthy of admission. In 1870, at Shadyside Hospital in Pittsburgh (then the Homeopathic Hospital), the Ladies' Charitable Association supported the care of indigents and decided who could stay at the institution at their expense. They said that they were "unwilling to pay for those who have brought themselves to distress by their own dissipation" M. Brignano, *Inheritors of a Glorious Reality, a History of Shadyside Hospital* (Pittsburgh: Shadyside Hospital, 1991), p. 29.

13. Rosenberg, *The Care of Strangers,* pp. 54–55.

14. Rosenberg, *The Care of Strangers,* pp. 341–347.

15. Stevens, R. *In Sickness and in Wealth* (New York: Basic Books, 1989), p. 96.

16. Rosenberg, *The Care of Strangers,* pp. 263, 278–282.

17. *Schloendorff v. Society of New York Hospital,* 211 N.Y. 125, 105 N.E. 92 (1914).

18. *Bing v. Thunig,* 2 N.Y. 656, 660–61, 163 N.Y.S.2d 3, 6, 143 N.E.2d 3, 4–5 (1957).

19. *Darling v. Charleston Community Memorial Hospital,* 33 Ill.2d 326, 211 N.E.2d 253 (1965).

20. *Darling,* 33 Ill. 2d 332, 211 N.E. 2d 257.

21. *Jackson v. Power,* 743 P.2d 1376 (Alaska 1987); see also L. B. Page, "Hospital Liability for Physicians: Widening National Quagmire," *Health Span,* July-Aug. 1989, p. 6.

Chapter Three

1. H. C. Sarvetnick, "Governance Responsibilities," *Issues in Health Care,* 1982, *3* (1), 76–80.

2. C. Houle, *Governing Boards: Their Nature and Nurture* (San Francisco: Jossey-Bass, 1989), p. 28.

3. R. Dimieri and S. Weiner, "The Public Interest and Governing Boards of Nonprofit Health Care Institutions," *Vanderbilt Law Review*, 1981, *34*, 1029, 1033–1034.

4. Kerr, "If Boards Mean Business," pp. 29, 30.

5. J. A. Witt, *Building a Better Hospital Board* (Ann Arbor, Mich.: Health Administration Press, 1987).

6. *Governance Issue Briefings* (Naperville, Ill.: Illinois Hospital Association, 1988), pp. 3.2–3.4.

7. R. L. Chandler, "Filling Empty Board Seats," *Hospital and Health Services Administration*, Winter 1980, pp. 69, 79–81.

8. W. Va. Code §16-5b-6a (1985).

9. *American Hospital Association v. Hansbarger*, 600 F.Supp. 465 (N.D.W.Va. 1984), aff'd, 783 F.2d 1184 (4th Cir. 1986).

10. *American Hospital Association v. Hansbarger*, 783 F.2d. 1184 (4th Cir. 1986).

11. L. Levy, "Reforming Board Reform," *Harvard Business Review*, Jan.-Feb. 1981, p. 166.

Chapter Four

1. P. F. Drucker, "What Business Can Learn from Nonprofits," *Harvard Business Review*, July-Aug. 1989, p. 88.

2. I.R.C. §501(c)(3) (1988).

3. Rev. Rul. 56-185, 1956-1 C.B. 202 (amended 1969).

4. Rev. Rul. 69-545, 1969-2 C.B. 117.

5. I.R.C. §501(b) (1988).

6. I.R.C. §501(e) (1988).

7. For a discussion of the adverse effects of Section 501(e) on shared hospital services, see J. P. McComb, Jr., "Supreme Court Tax Ruling Impedes Forming of Hospital Shared Services," *Modern Health Care*, July 1981, p. 100.

8. *Medical Center of Vermont, Inc. v. City of Burlington*, 356 A.2d 1352 (Vt. 1989).

9. *Utah County v. Intermountain Health Care*, 709 P.2d 265 (1985).

10. Clark, R. C., "Does the Nonprofit Form Fit the Hospital Industry?," *Harvard Law Review*, 1980, *93*, 1416–1417.
11. Dimieri and Weiner, "The Public Interest," pp. 1033–1034.
12. Herzlinger, R. E., and Krasker, W. S. "Who Profits from Nonprofits?," *Harvard Business Review*, Jan.-Feb. 1987, p. 93.

Chapter Five

1. J. D. Harvey, "Evaluating the Performance of the Chief Executive Officer," *Hospital and Health Services Administration*, Spring 1978, pp. 5, 6.

Chapter Six

1. Joint Commission on Accreditation of Healthcare Organizations, *Accreditation Manual for Hospitals* (Chicago: Joint Commission on Accreditation of Healthcare Organizations, 1990), G.B. 1.2.4.5, p. 47 [hereafter *Accreditation Manual*].
2. R. L. Johnson, "Appraising Performance at the Top," *Hospital and Health Services Administration*, Fall 1987, p. 36.
3. *Accreditation Manual*, G.B. 1.21, p. 50.
4. B. S. Bader, R. J. Umbdenstock, and W. M. Hageman, *Board Self-Evaluation Manual* (Rockville, Md.: Bader & Associates, 1986).

Chapter Seven

1. *Stern v. Lucy Webb Hayes Nat'l Training School for Deaconesses and Missionaries*, 381 F.Supp. 1003 (S.D.N.Y. 1974).
2. *Stern*, 381 F. Supp. 1013–14.
3. Stevens, *In Sickness and in Wealth*, p. 327.
4. See Conditions of Participation for Hospitals, 42 C.F.R. §482 (1989).

5. Pub. L. No. 93-641, 88 Stat. 2226 (1975) (codified as amended at 42 U.S.C.A. §300k-t (West 1982 & Supp. 1990)).

6. Established in 1950 by the American College of Surgeons as the Joint Commission on Accreditation of Hospitals, JCAHO is now sponsored by several medical bodies, including the American Hospital Association and the American Medical Association. It provides inspection and accreditation for hospitals and recently has begun to provide the same voluntary services to health maintenance organizations and home health care groups.

7. See W. Bogdanich, "Small Comfort: Prized by Hospitals, Accreditation Hides Perils Patients Face," *Wall Street Journal,* Oct. 12, 1988, p. A1.

8. Sherman Antitrust Act, ch. 647, §1, 26 Stat. 209, 209 (1890) (codified as amended at 15 U.S.C.A. §2 (West 1973 and Supp. 1990)).

9. Sherman Antitrust Act, ch. 647, §2, 26 Stat. 209, 209 (1890) (codified as amended at 15 U.S.C.A. §2 (West 1973 and Supp. 1990)).

10. Clayton Act, ch. 323, §2, 38 Stat. 730, 730–31 (1914) (codified as amended at 15 U.S.C.A. §13 (West 1973)).

11. A tying arrangement conditions the sale of one product (the tying product) on the purchase of a second product (the tied product) primarily to prevent the purchaser from buying the tied product from the seller's competitor. A requirements contract commits a buyer to purchase all of his needs of a specified product for a given time period from the seller to supply all of the buyer's needs, or both.

12. Clayton Act, ch. 323, §3, 38 Stat. 730, 731 (1914) (codified as amended at 15 U.S.C.A. §14 (West 1973)).

13. Federal Trade Commission Act, ch. 311, §5, 38 Stat. 717, 718 (1914) (codified as amended at 15 U.S.C.A. §45 (West 1973 & Supp. 1990)).

14. *Goldfarb v. Virginia State Bar,* 421 U.S. 773 (1975).

15. *Hospital Building Co. v. Trustees of Rex Hospital,* 425 U.S. 738 (1976).

Chapter Eight

1. Hospital Survey and Construction Act, ch. 958, 60 Stat. 1040 (1946) (codified as amended in scattered sections of 24, 33, 42, 46, 48 and 49 U.S.C.A.).
2. Hospital Trustee Association of Pennsylvania, *The Board and Strategic Planning*, Trustee Folio 10 (1985).
3. N. McMillan, *Planning for Survival: A Handbook for Hospital Trustees*, 2nd ed. (Chicago: American Hospital Publishing, 1985), p. 95.
4. See L. R. Fritz, "The Mission Statement: Framework for the Hospital's Strategic Plan," *Trustee*, July 1989, pp. 8–9, 25.
5. A. Flexner, *Medical Education in the United States and Canada: A Report to the Carnegie Foundation for the Advancement of Teaching* (Boston: D. B. Updike, The Merrymount Press, 1910).
6. Stevens, *In Sickness and in Wealth*, pp. 61–66.

Chapter Nine

1. J. A. Alexander, *Current Issues in Governance*, pamphlet (Chicago: Hospital Research and Education Trust, 1986), p. 5.
2. Stevens, *In Sickness and in Wealth*, p. 45.
3. S. Law, *Blue Cross: What Went Wrong* (New Haven, CT: Yale University Press, 1974), p. 11.
4. Health Insurance for the Aged Act, Pub. L. No. 89-97, tit. I, 79 Stat. 290, 310-80 (1965) (codified as amended at 42 U.S.C.A. §1395 et seq. (West 1983 and Supp. 1990)).
5. Ernst & Whinney, *Introduction to Health Care for New Hospital Trustees*, 1988, pp. 111–112.
6. American Institute of Certified Public Accountants, *Hospital Audit Guide* (New York: American Institute of Certified Public Accountants, 1972).
7. MedisGroups is a software system owned and marketed by MediQual Systems, Inc., of Westborough, Mass. The system tries to determine severity of illness by utilizing 260

key clinical findings to produce admission scores from 0 through 4. These indicate increasing risk of organ failure.

8. For a helpful guide in this area, see J. Elrod and J. Wilkinson, *Hospital Project Financing and Refinancing Under Prospective Payment* (Chicago: American Hospital Publishing, 1985).

9. American Hospital Association, *Hospital Capital Finance,* First Quarter, 1986, p. 4.

Chapter Ten

1. Joint Commission on Accreditation of Healthcare Organizations, *Risk Management and Quality Assurance: Issues and Interactions* (Chicago: Joint Commission on Accreditation of Healthcare Organizations, 1986), p. 5 [hereafter *Risk Management*].

2. *Accreditation Manual,* M.S. 5.2.1, p. 109.

3. *Accreditation Manual,* Q.A. 1, p. 211.

4. *Accreditation Manual,* Q.A. 1, p. 211.

5. Hospital Trustee Association of Pennsylvania, *Keys to Better Hospital Governance Through Better Information* (Camp Hill, Pa.: Hospital Trustee Association of Pennsylvania, 1983) [hereafter *Keys to Better Governance*].

6. *Keys to Better Governance,* p. 11.

7. *Keys to Better Governance,* p. 53.

8. *Risk Management,* p. 5.

9. J. E. Orlikoff and G. B. Lanham, "Why Risk Management and Quality Assurance Should Be Integrated," *Hospitals,* June 1, 1981, p. 54.

10. *Accreditation Manual,* Q.A. 1.3, p. 211.

11. Presentation by James E. Orlikoff, Pennsylvania Hospital Trustee Association Fall Conference, Oct. 19, 1988.

12. D. M. Berwick, "Continuous Improvement as an Ideal in Health Care," *New England Journal of Medicine,* 1989, *320,* 53.

13. W. R. Fifer, "Is There a New Paradigm for Quality Management?," *Quality Letter for Healthcare Leaders,* Sept. 1989, p. 16.

14. *Accreditation Manual,* M.S. 3.5, p. 102.
15. *Accreditation Manual,* M.S. 3.5, p. 102.
16. *Accreditation Manual,* M.S. 2.1, p. 98.
17. *Keys To Better Governance* has indicated that, at least in the quality assurance area, board responsibility includes resolving quality issues between hospital management and the medical staff that cannot be resolved at a lower level. Unfortunately, no mechanism for accomplishing this resolution is suggested. See *Keys to Better Governance,* pp. 52–53.
18. *Darling,* 33 Ill.2d 326, 211 N.E.2d 253 (1965).
19. *Patrick v. Burgett,* 486 U.S. 97 (1988).
20. Pub. L. No. 99-660, §§401-32, 100 Stat. 3743, 3784–94 (1986) (current version 42 U.S.C.A. §§11101–52 (West Supp. 1990)).
21. *Stern v. Lucy Webb Hayes Nat'l Training School for Deaconesses and Missionaries,* 381 F.Supp. 1003 (S.D.N.Y. 1974).
22. For discussions of physician membership on the hospital governing board, see C. M. Ewell, "Hospital-Loyal Physicians Can Bring Benefits to Boards," *Modern Healthcare,* Jan. 27, 1989, p. 32; M. Dreuth and S. Blau, "Physicians in Hospital Governance," *Trustee,* Aug. 1988, p. 24.
23. Peer Review Improvement Act of 1982, Pub. L. No. 97-248, §§141-150, 99 Stat. 324, 381-195 (1982) (current version in scattered sections of 42 U.S.C.A. §§1305–1396 (1983 and Supp. 1990)).
24. S. E. Kellie and J. T. Kelly, "Medicare Peer Review Organization Preprocedure Review Criteria," *Journal of the American Medical Association,* 1991, *265* (10), 1265–1270, 1266.

Chapter Eleven

1. Alexander, *Current Issues in Governance,* p. 5. For a more detailed discussion of restructuring, see J. P. McComb, Jr., *One Trustee Looks at the Restructured Hospital System* (Camp Hill, Pa.: Hospital Trustee Association of Pennsylvania, 1986).

2. *Erie v. The Hamot Medical Center*, No. 138-A-1989 *aff'd*, No. 1319 C.D. 1990 and No. 1320 C.D. 1990 (PA Cmwlth, Jan. 9, 1992).

3. See also *Utah County v. Intramountain Health Care*, 709 P.2d 265 (Ut. 1985), and *Medical Center of Vermont v. City of Burlington*, 566 A. 2d 1352 (Vt. 1989).

Chapter Twelve

1. Pub. L. No. 93-641, 88 Stat. 2220 (1975) (codified as amended at 42 U.S.C.A. §§300k–t (West 1982 & Supp. 1990)).

2. 42 U.S.C.A., 300 K-2(2).

3. 42 U.S.C.A., 300 K-2(5).

4. 42 U.S.C.A., 300 K-2(7).

5. Stevens, *In Sickness and in Wealth*, p. 61.

6. H. S. Zuckerman, *Multi-Institutional Hospital Systems* (Chicago: Hospital Research and Educational Trust, 1979); see also Hospital Research and Educational Trust, *Multi-Hospital Systems: Policy Issues for the Future* (Chicago: Hospital Research and Educational Trust, 1981).

7. J. Greene, "2 VHA Execs Quit; Restructuring Eyed," *Modern Healthcare*, Sept. 16, 1988, p. 4.

8. A. T. Solovy, "Shopping for an Alliance: Your Business Plan Is Key," *Trustee*, Dec. 1988, p. 8.

9. G. L. McManis, "Not-for-Profit Alliances Need to Focus on Value," *Modern Healthcare*, Oct. 13, 1989, p. 40.

10. P. J. Kenkel, "Meeting the Challenge of Managed Care in Hospitals," *Modern Healthcare*, Nov. 17, 1989, pp. 52–53.

11. H. R. Berry, "Managed Care's 4th Generation," *Group Practice Journal*, July-Aug. 1989, p. 1.

Chapter Thirteen

1. See Alexander, *Current Issues in Governance*, p. 1.

2. Stevens, *In Sickness and in Wealth*, p. 38.

3. Stevens, *In Sickness and in Wealth*, p. 38.

4. Stevens, *In Sickness and in Wealth*, p. 364.
5. At the AHA, some members (for example, nonprofit and investor-owned hospitals) may have antithetical views on policy development.
6. See Coddington, Keen, Moore, and Clarke, *The Crisis in Health Care*, for further discussion.

Index

171